LOOKING AFTER YOUR
NUTS&
BOLTS

LOOKING AFTER YOUR
NUTS&
BOLTS

PHIL GIFFORD'S
KIWI MEN'S
HEALTH GUIDE

A catalogue record for this book is available from the
National Library of New Zealand

ISBN 978-1-927262-48-1

An Upstart Press Book
Published in 2017 by Upstart Press Ltd
Level 4, 15 Huron St, Takapuna 0622
Auckland, New Zealand

Cover designed by redinc.
Printed by 1010 Printing International Ltd., China

While every effort has been made to ensure all the material contained in this book
is correct and up to date, the author and the publishers cannot be held liable for the
information. Readers should always consult their medical practitioners.

Photo Credits
Richard Redgrove: 24.
Getty Images: 83, 153, 176.

This book is dedicated to the men who bravely told their own health stories, some of them deeply personal, in the hope that their experiences might encourage their brothers in arms to stay healthy.

Contents

Foreword

When my good mate Phil rang and asked me if I would do the foreword for this book I'd just arrived home from a tour to Britain with the Kiwis league team. It was a sadly appropriate time. My wife had just broken the news to me that my eldest brother Jack had been diagnosed with prostate cancer.

My other brother Gary died of bladder cancer, and he could have possibly been alive today if he'd gone to the doctor sooner.

I've been a campaigner for men's health for some time. I'm the patron of Prostate Cancer New Zealand and several other great health organisations.

Why? Because too many men die of ill health for a very simple reason: they don't go to the doctor.

The other thing is that if you do go to the doctor, and you're not satisfied with the diagnosis, go to another doctor and get a second opinion. As much as I admire doctors, they're not all-seeing. One may not always pick something up; something that another may rapidly find.

I've been very fortunate in that when I developed a rare form of prostate cancer both my doctor, Bruce Page, and my oncologist, Robin Smart, were quick to recognise the problem, and to treat it.

As you can see, men's health is a very personal issue to me, as ill health has affected both my brothers.

It's an honour to be involved with a book that aims to help brothers from our wider family, all Kiwi blokes, to lead longer, healthier and happier lives.

Sir Peter Leitch, KNZM, QSM

Thanks

This book would not have been possible without the help of some wonderful people.

I'm deeply grateful to Graeme Washer, my doctor and a friend, who was unfailingly positive and helpful, from the time we first discussed the idea to his final proofreading of the manuscript. Please take the time to check out an organisation very dear to his and my heart, the Men's Health Trust New Zealand.

Their website is menshealthnz.org.nz.

My thanks for the patience and encouragement offered by Kevin and Warren at Upstart Press, who were always generous-spirited when, for various reasons, the delivery date for the book was set back several times.

My wife Jan, as she has since my first full book in 1990, was the first to read chapters as they were finished. My love and thanks to her for her patience when her worthwhile suggestions weren't always immediately welcomed, and for sharing the humour when we both realised we were starting to suspect we had the symptoms described in whatever chapter we were poring over.

A huge thank you to the non-medical people who so freely and generously offered their time, expertise and talents. To Sir Peter Leitch, Nic Gill, Lee-Anne Wann, Paul Thomas, Jim Eagles, Mike Chunn, Leigh Hart, Paul Ego, Phil Kingsley Jones, Jeremy Corbett and Dai Henwood, you're all champions.

I was constantly amazed at the good-hearted way all the hugely busy medical specialists I spoke to not only gave up their time to be interviewed, but took even more time to carefully edit early drafts to make sure that what was said was accurate. It was slightly staggering too that they were all happy to carefully pass on, in terms a medical ignoramus like me could understand, the wisdom they've accumulated over a lifetime of skilled work.

Phil Gifford, Auckland, January 2017

No Kale Smoothies

The book you're holding now isn't going to suggest a switch to silverbeet sandwiches, organic oat bran enemas, kale smoothies, or naked sweat lodge fasting.

In the words of Billy Connolly, 'What's the point in adding three years to your life if you're bloody miserable in all the years before them?'

What's being offered here is a place to check out ideas that could help you live not just longer, but better. You won't be invited to buy pills, potions, pamphlets, magnets, or miracle fitness machines.

Everyone who's quoted is an expert, whether it's the fitness trainer who guides the All Blacks, or the surgeon who does prostate checks more often than Winston Peters sneaks a look in a mirror.

So what are my credentials for writing this book?

One. I've been a male all my life.

Two. I've jumped, sometimes staggered, through all the usual lifetime hoops. Marriage, fatherhood, divorce and remarriage. In the workplace, I've been hired, sacked, resigned, been sued and counter-sued. Owned houses, sold houses, moved houses. Lived in the country, lived in the city.

Three. I've made a living writing and talking since I was 18. I've never believed in a book as much as I believe in this one.

Four. I've got skin in the health game. Both hips replaced, prostate cancer, bowel cancer, skin cancer, but happily now very much, as Willie Nelson says, 'standing upright on the ground'.

With time, you grow to realise women are smarter about how they look after their health. Does anyone think retirement villages are full of more women than men by accident? At the last count, in 2015, New Zealand Statistics said Kiwi women live nearly four years longer than Kiwi men (83.2 years compared to 79.5 years).

Talking with friends it became clear guys aren't big on asking health questions. Even if they have the time it somehow doesn't feel right. A mate has to have a heart attack before we find out what the early symptoms are. The first thing on a guy's mind in a doctor's office is how soon he can get out.

The aim in these pages is simple. You can find out what you need to know, and have some fun in the process. Billy Connolly's right, there's no need to be bloody miserable along the way.

User's Note: At the end of many chapters in this book there are website addresses for reputable local organisations dealing with health. Feel free to Google for more health details elsewhere but, be warned, to discover an area swarming with snake oil salesmen and tinfoil hat-wearing fanatics, just search the web for 'disease alternative cures'.

Your Prostate
An Annoying Little Bugger

For something as small as a walnut, your prostate can be an annoying little bugger, but it doesn't have to get the better of you.

It lurks inside your body behind your penis, and gets heavily involved in your sex life, helping it when you're young, being a potential nuisance when you're olwder.

When you're a kid and hair starts to grow in funny places, your prostate's growing too. Just for fun, it'll eventually screw up how you pee.

At primary school, you and your mates can pee over a fence. By your late teens you'll hit the middle of it. By the time you're getting a pension the good old prostate will probably make you glad if you can even spray the base.

To really keep you on your toes, a prostate is also a fertile breeding ground for cancer. By the time a man is in his 80s, there's a good chance he'll have prostate cancer; although, in that case, it's unlikely he'll die from it.

The good news? Prostate cancer, detected early, is a disease that can definitely be cured.

Your GP and your family tree are your first lines of defence in making sure it doesn't sneak up on you. Your general practitioner will probably be looking at checking your prostate from the age of 50.

Visiting a GP, says Auckland urologist Chris Hawke, isn't something that should be left until things go very badly. 'A guy is far more likely to die of a heart attack or a stroke than he is of prostate cancer, but he should be getting all these things managed.'

In the case of prostate cancer, like all diseases, finding out early is way better than finding out late. Regularly visiting your doctor for a general check-up can be a lifesaving idea.

A slightly odd twist with prostate cancer is that some of the symptoms are very similar to the annoying, but largely harmless, issue of an enlarged prostate, which can make it hard to urinate, and/or make it necessary to pee numerous times during the day and night.

There's also the possibility there won't be any symptoms at all, which makes a regular check-up by your doctor or a specialist an even better idea.

Shaking the family tree is important too. 'If your dad, your brother, your uncle, some sort of first-degree male relative had prostate cancer then maybe you should be checked as early as 40,' says Chris Hawke.

'If you have a family history of prostate cancer it certainly should be earlier than 50. There is definitely a familial element with prostate cancer. It's not as clear cut a genetic picture as it is with breast cancer. But we know some of the genes that put you at high risk for prostate cancer.'

So what exactly is a prostate anyway? And what does it actually do?

It's a small gland between your bladder and your penis. Your urethra, the tube that carries urine from your bladder to your penis, passes right through the middle of the prostate.

When the prostate is healthy, its main role is to make a fluid that protects sperm. Remember we mentioned its involvement in your sex life?

So far, so straightforward. Where things get trickier is what happens when it grows with age. Before puberty the prostate isn't developed, which makes it much easier to urinate. Nothing's squeezing the urethra.

One of life's realities is that past a certain age a prostate will become enlarged. 'Everyone's prostate gets larger as they get older,' says Chris. 'It's very common. Your hair will fall out and go grey, and you'll get a bigger prostate. You can pretty much take it to the bank.

'From the prostate enlargement point of view, the things that guys start to notice is that they start getting up a couple of times at night to pee, then three times at night, and then not getting much sleep. Getting up at least once a night as you get older sort of becomes par for the course.

'Then it starts to intrude on their day. They start to know where every toilet is around town. They have to stop a game of golf or whatever and go and have a pee. It's getting slower, harder to start, trickles away, all those things, which are usually a sign of a benign non-cancerous enlarged prostate.'

So far, so harmless. An enlarged prostate can usually be treated with medication, with drugs that make the prostate muscle relax. Side effects are quite minor.

What's the difference between the symptoms of an enlarged prostate and prostate cancer? Not a lot. By and large the signs are not blindingly obvious. There might be blood in your urine. If there is, don't mess around. 'That,' says Chris, 'can be anything from a kidney stone to a growth on the kidney, often cancerous, to an enlarged prostate to a bladder tumour. Get it checked.'

If there are no neon signs, how does a doctor work out whether you've got prostate cancer? There will almost certainly be the snap of a rubber glove. Medically it's called a digital examination. Another phrase would be a finger in your butt. Embarrassing? Probably. Essential? Of course. It's the quickest and most sure way for a doctor to find out if your prostate is very enlarged, and whether there are signs of cancer on the exterior.

(I spoke at a national urologists' conference in Hamilton in 2011. If you don't look forward to a digital exam it turns out neither do they. In conversation with a very experienced urologist, he said, 'Keep in mind we're not enjoying the situation either. Although I guess you do get used to it. They say the first 20,000 are the worst.')

Your doctor may arrange for you to get a blood sample for a PSA test.

The letters PSA can mean a disease that affects kiwifruit vines,

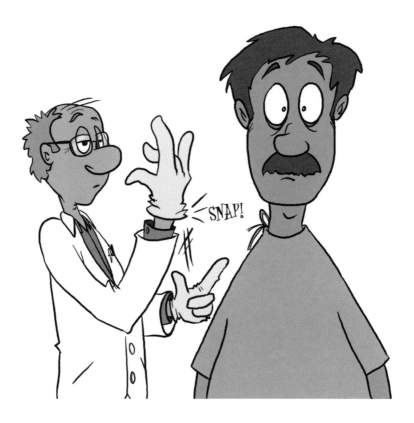

or stand for the Public Service Association, New Zealand's biggest union. But in the world of the prostate it stands for prostate specific antigen, a protein produced by the prostate. Changing levels can be a sign there are cancer cells in your prostate.

Medically, PSA also stands for controversy. Argument has raged for several years over whether PSA tests have led to men having procedures they didn't really need to have. It's an argument likely to go on for some time. In 2010 *New York Times* writer Dana Jennings, who, after PSA testing and extensive surgery, was found to have an extremely aggressive form of cancer that sprang from prostate cancer, wrote about studies suggesting prostate cancer in men was being overtreated.

He said, 'My biggest problem with the studies — and, of course, this is the nature of such studies — is that they reduce me and all my brothers-in-disease to abstractions, to cancer-bearing ciphers. Among those dry words, we are not living, breathing and terrified men, but merely our prostate cancers, whether slow or bold.'

In 2010 I was being treated for prostate cancer, and, asked to write a story about the experience for the *Sunday Star-Times*, said, 'I'm halfway through a treatment involving radioactive seeds in the prostate, and, to put it bluntly, am bloody glad I have the opportunity to do so. To me the choice between taking a chance that my tumours may never threaten my life, and having them treated, was simple. Treatment first, daylight second.'

My cancer was at a stage where it needed attention. But that may not be the case for everyone. How does that work?

As Chris Hawke explains, the longer you live, the more chance there is you'll have some form of prostate cancer, but there's a good chance it won't be what you die of.

'We know that if you do autopsies on men in their 80s who have died of other causes,' he says, 'about half of them also have prostate cancer. So it becomes very common. You could make similar arguments about other organs in the body. They become progressively more diseased.

'One in 10 guys will be aware of prostate cancer in his life. One in three of those guys die of it.'

For those of you, like me, who flunked maths at school, here's how that works. Put 100 Kiwi men in a room and 10 of them will be diagnosed with prostate cancer in their lifetime. So 90 leave the room unscathed. Of the 10 that are left, three, sadly, will die. Seven will walk out after treatment.

Of the unlucky three, the fatal problem will be that the prostate cancer has spread before it has been detected and treated.

Hormone treatment can extend life if that happens. The less testosterone the testicles are producing the better. But it's not a cure.

'The length of time prostate cancer responds to hormone treatment is anything from a year or two if you're unlucky,' says Chris, 'through to 10 years, if you're very lucky. But eventually what we now know is that the cancer cells start to be able to produce their own hormones, and eventually not having any testosterone doesn't help any more. The cancer starts to grow back, and spreads.

'It's never been a disease which is particularly responsive to chemotherapy. Even the 21st-century chemotherapy drugs we have for prostate cancer will only reduce symptoms, and extend your period of survival, although not by much. No one has ever been cured of prostate cancer with chemo.'

Nevertheless, in the last five years many specialists have decided that in some cases, if a cancer is picked up at an early enough stage, there may be no need for immediate treatment, especially if you're in your 50s or 60s.

Chris explains. 'It became obvious over the years that with PSA screening we were picking up some cancers at such an early stage that they probably were insignificant. In a lot of cases, we could keep a guy under surveillance for maybe five or 10 years, which means that he doesn't have to put up with any side effects of treatment. So surveillance is something which has really become quite a common option in the last five years.'

What's actually involved with surveillance? Blood tests on a regular basis to check PSA, the rubber-gloved finger once a year, and about every two years a biopsy, where tiny samples are taken from your prostate. A biopsy is uncomfortable, but not painful.

On the other hand, if you're older when the cancer is detected, or it's at a more advanced stage, there are two directions for treatment: one is radiotherapy, the other is surgery.

Radiotherapy can be applied in two ways. Brachytherapy involves putting radioactive seeds right into the tumour in your prostate. The tumour is scanned, and mapped, and then about 100 tiny seeds are injected by needles into the prostate through your backside. (If that sounds deeply unpleasant, it's all done under anaesthetic, and when you wake up, and spend a night in hospital to get over the anaesthetic, there's no pain at all.)

Brachytherapy is not just used for prostate cancer. It has traditionally been used for cervical cancer and, to a smaller degree, for liver cancer. The seeds are tiny canisters — like little pellets of titanium with radioactive iodine inside.

How do they work? Radiation damages DNA within the nucleus of cancer cells. The cancer cells have to try to repair themselves and, thankfully, a cancer cell is usually nowhere near as good at that as a normal cell.

Back home, are you now walking around with a glowing groin so radioactive North Korea would be interested in strapping you to a long-range missile? No. The types of radioactive isotopes used decay over a short period of time. Only the harmless titanium pellets that encase the iodine are with you forever.

'If an archaeologist is digging you up in 1000 years' time,' says Chris Hawke, 'he or she will be thinking, "What are these pellets?"'

But the archaeologist will be in no danger. Iodine isotope has a two-month half-life. In other words, you get half the radiation dose in the first two months. The dose left in the pellets halves again after another two months. By the time a year comes up, you have about 1% of the energy left in the pellets, and can pretty much forget about them.

External radiotherapy has the same effect on cancer cells' DNA as brachytherapy, but does have the disadvantage of having to pass through healthy tissue on the way to the prostate.

'The technology has improved substantially in the last 10 years to really aim that radiation a lot more accurately,' says Chris Hawke, 'but you still can't get away from the fact that the tissues that are cheek by jowl against the prostate, notably the rectum and the floor of the bladder, are going to get a dose of radiation.'

You may not be a candidate for radiotherapy. The option then is surgery.

'People get a bit confused,' says Chris, 'because a lot of surgery we do, in fact the majority, is of an endoscopic nature, what is often called a rebore.'

The squeamish should possibly look away now, but remember the operation is conducted with a full anaesthetic. 'We use a telescope up through the penis, into the middle of the prostate, and core it out, so that a guy can pass urine more easily.

'That doesn't solve any cancer issues because you are leaving at least half the prostate, a shell of tissue, behind. Most prostate cancer grows towards the outer part of the prostate, so if there was cancer there, you'd be leaving most of the cancer behind if you do a rebore.

'If a guy has got a really big prostate, is having a lot of difficulty passing urine, only just getting by, and has cancer in his prostate, you are better off operating on his prostate and taking it out. You will solve his urinary difficulties as well as getting the cancer out all in the one go.

'So to deal with cancer by operating you have got to take out the entire prostate, and that means you have literally got a gap between the floor of the bladder and the urethra tube. So you have got to join those two things back together, to give the urine a path to come out.'

Expect some problems holding urine back for a couple of months after having the whole prostate taken out. Thankfully normal control returns in about 90% of cases after a few months.

What about sex? Not as bad as the occasional water cooler gossip might have it.

Whether it's brachytherapy or an operation, there is damage done to nerves that run through the pelvis and along the base of the penis. With brachytherapy there's a dose of radiation to those nerves. With surgery they'll be bruised or stretched.

What happens to the ability to have an erection is usually different, depending on whether you've had radiotherapy or an operation.

With brachytherapy there's often a delayed reaction. After a few years, the difficulty in having an erection that age usually produces anyway may speed up. (By the way, despite the propaganda Hugh

Hefner's publicity people spread about his sexual prowess in his 80s, tell-all books by the girls he lives with suggest he's not so much a raging bull in the bedroom as a tired old voyeuristic steer gazing over the fence. Hate to break the news, but a man in his 80s is unlikely to be a 'twice a night and three times on Sunday' guy in the sack.)

With surgery, the pattern of sexual performance gradually dwindling with time is turned on its head with initial problems followed, in many cases, by slow, progressive recovery.

In either case, surgery or radiotherapy, there are various kinds of medical help to restore your sex life after prostate treatment. It may be drugs; it may be a vacuum pump; it may be injections. Your surgeon will have recommendations if you want them.

The only prostate operation that unfortunately guarantees no more erections is when a man has high-risk cancer, which has spread outside the edge of the prostate, and a surgeon has to go wider, with what's called a wide local resection.

In that case, you're really making a choice between your erection or your life. 'You don't want to leave cancer behind for the sake of sparing erectile nerves,' says Chris Hawke. 'Not much point in having the best erection in the graveyard!'

To sum up, as with all diseases, early treatment will always be better than discovering prostate cancer late.

'That's the modern face of prostate cancer,' says Chris. 'You go along to see your GP for a general check, or something is bothering you. You have a GP who is proactive. They check a few things and they find something is amiss. Most commonly the PSA is up.

'You get sent along to a urologist, there are more investigations, the cancer is discovered, hopefully at an early stage, you get treatment, and you live to see your grandkids grow up.'

You'll find the extensive Prostate Cancer Foundation of New Zealand site at prostate.org.nz.

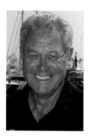

PJ Montgomery

As the international voice of yachting, PJ Montgomery is never lost for words. From 'the America's Cup is now New Zealand's Cup' to describing waves in the Southern Ocean as 'the liquid Himalayas', he's always found the right phrase. But when he was told in 2006 he had tested positive for prostate cancer he was basically struck dumb. He shares his story in the hope other men won't put themselves through the distress he imposed on himself.

I'd had various issues with my waterworks and bladder in 2006, so I went to my GP, John Mayhew. It was common garden stuff, preventative maintenance. I was at an age in my mid-40s when I needed to start being checked.

But checking out the bladder issues involves a bit more than what a GP would usually do, so John Mayhew sent me to urologist Michael Mackey.

My PSA (blood test) was good but not that good. A finger up the butt was really the answer. So I said to Michael Mackey, 'Well, if you insist.' He did insist and, as a result of the procedure, Michael requested I get a biopsy done. He inspected my prostate and took some time. Michael then explained one side of my prostate was hard so he wanted to check further.

I was booked for a 'transrectal ultrasound guided prostate biopsy' for Monday 12 June 2006. Michael told me he had found something quite crustaceous and that was when he decided to get the biopsy done.

The biopsy confirmed what he felt. On Monday 19 June I went back to see Michael. He said it looked serious and he had some bad news. The biopsy of the right lobe of the prostate was positive. He was trying to tell me I had cancer. He said if I was 10 or certainly 15 years older he'd do nothing.

What I seized on was there were some guys who live into their

80s with it. That every man by the time he's in his 80s probably has prostate cancer, but it hasn't developed enough that it becomes what he dies of.

So did I just hear white noise once Michael had said 'cancer' and 'positive'? I think I did. I was shocked. He told me what I had, but I think it was 'whoomph'. It was the shock of it that meant the message didn't register. It just went over me. I didn't digest it. I went into denial.

I just wasn't being realistic and was really living a lie. At home, with my dear wife Claudia, I downplayed the news. The only person I told I had cancer was my physiotherapist David Abercrombie, and he told me in very blunt terms that I should do something about it. Every week David told me in frank, blunt language that I was being stupid and staying in denial would not solve anything

But I found excuses to not do anything. My urologist, Michael, was going to France to ride in the L'Étape du Tour, a stage that amateurs are able to ride during the Tour de France.

I do remember thinking, 'Well, Michael's going away so that takes the heat off.' I knew he was away for four to six weeks. So I went home and did nothing.

The more I recall it I know I would have thought about it several times a day. Not once a day. To the point where I was thinking, 'Have I really got it? How bad is it?'

I do recall the torture I was going through. Am I living a lie or do I have time on my side? Then the cloud lifted . . . In mid-August, two months after my diagnosis, Michael Mackey's wonderful practice nurse Janine Pinfold phoned and left a message on our home phone. In the message, Janine said they were worried they had not heard from me and time was becoming important.

The message was picked up by Claudia. For the first time, she realised the situation was not as sunny as my actions, or lack of them, suggested.

In mid-August I went back to Doc Mayhew and told him about

my visits to Michael Mackey and my stupid reaction and how I was in denial. Doc Mayhew was fantastic and gave me some excellent questions to ask Michael. When I left Doc I was in no doubt I had to get real and that living in denial meant I would not be living much longer.

On 1 September Claudia came with me to an appointment with Michael. My first question was, 'Michael, have I really got cancer?' He looked at me, and I've never forgotten it, as if to say, 'Am I looking at a dimwit here?' He said, 'I've told you that.' That was the problem. I wouldn't accept it.

I asked another couple of questions. Then Claudia took over, conducted the orchestra, and did the talking. I just sat there. The appointments were made.

Action was taken and an operation would happen within the next fortnight. This was serious and now needed urgent attention.

When we left I can remember the relief of knowing something was happening. My own conscience was relieved that action was finally being taken. I did get the message in the end. Fortunately, the cancer was confined to my prostate. The big issue was that if I messed around for too long it could spread into my lymph nodes, and then I'd be in real trouble. While I still had a lot of apprehension, once it was out in the open there was a weight off my shoulders.

Back in June, Michael had given me a book to read, *Prostate and Cancer* by Sheldon Marks, which I've still got in my bedside drawer. I'd taken it home and never bothered to look at it. After our September meeting I read it and considered the options. I went for the operation.

Claudia and I were going to Edinburgh in September. We cancelled everything. On 13 September 2006, less than a fortnight from the crucial meeting with Michael, I was being operated on.

Once the cloud lifted, I had a very supportive wife and family and the burden was shared. Claudia was fantastic. I went to Ascot Hospital for the operation and she was there in all my waking time.

We already had a fantastic relationship, but I think our marriage was strengthened during this time. I learned the hard way that you need to share.

(Happily, the operation was a success and regular checks confirm that, 10 years later, there is no reccurrence of the disease.)

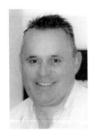

Justin Worsley

Justin Worsley is a 48-year-old business development manager for the Laser Group, a national network of plumbers and electricians. Self-employed for 20 years, he develops franchises for Laser throughout New Zealand, travelling every second or third week. When he was 46, he was diagnosed with prostate cancer.

I've been reasonably good at having regular health checks for the last 20-odd years. Back in my late 20s I had to go to the doctor for an insurance policy health check. Out of that it came back that I had high cholesterol. So that started me on the journey of having regular checks.

It normally comes every February, after my birthday; it was always a birthday present to myself, to get in and see the doc and have a health check.

As it happens, when the prostate cancer was detected, I'd gone in to see my GP to try to get rid of the back end of a chest infection and a cold. I happened to have quite a busy time coming up and I thought I want to see my doctor and get some antibiotics and get it cleared up, I don't want it hanging around.

In the conversation, I said, 'By the way Doc, when was the last time I had my health check?' He said, 'You didn't come this year (meaning the previous February), so it will be about 18 months.' I said, 'Give me the blood test. I'd better go and have it.' And so I did. That started the ball rolling, I suppose.

After the test he told me my cholesterol had crept up a little but, more importantly, my PSA level, last time we checked it, was around about 2.5 or 3 (nothing out of the norm) but it had now gone to 6.5.

He said we'd check it again in two or three months. I had forgotten about it and then, all of a sudden, you know it is reasonably serious when a letter arrives in your letter box from your doctor saying give me a call urgently. So he was onto it.

He said you need to get in and have that second lot of blood tests; it has been a couple of months. During that time my PSA level had gone from 6.5 to 8.5, so things were starting to escalate quite quickly.

I went in and had the blood tests again. I changed my diet at that time, I had moved towards a paleo, high-protein-type diet. I'd done a bit of research and found that a change in diet could have an effect on PSA readings, so I wasn't totally convinced. I thought it might be an artificial reading.

My doctor said to phone Chris Hawke, a urologist. I said, 'Give me some time over Christmas. I'll move away from red meat towards fish and chicken and see if it makes any difference.' A bit of avoidance really.

But in late January the tests came back exactly the same and I went to see Chris.

The first thing I had was a magnetic resonance imaging scan. The MRI identified that there was something there. We didn't quite know what, but there was something showing up within the prostate.

Then I went back in about a week or two after the MRI and had the biopsy. I was told it is pretty aggressive, it is real, you've got to deal with it and these are your options.

I decided to go for the full removal. Because of my age, the challenge was if I had radiation therapy and the cancer came back in about 10 years' time, I would only be in my late 50s and at that age it is a lot harder to deal with. So having my prostate removed made a lot of sense. There were some issues that came with it, but it was the best decision.

There weren't many side effects. I think it is probably because of my age (being younger than most prostate cancer sufferers). I went back and spoke to Chris afterwards and said, 'How many guys my age do you deal with a year?' He said, 'I'd be lucky if I deal with one or two.' That surprised me.

I bounced back reasonably quickly. Within a month to five weeks I no longer needed to use pads for incontinence. That was pretty good. And then, obviously, the other side of it, the sexual function, I think I was back up to 70% within two to three months and it has slowly gotten better from there. It wasn't too bad.

Since the operation, I've been every three months for blood tests.

There were two types of surgery that Chris could have done, and the one we chose was the full open me up and have a good look around and take the prostate out.

The reason for that was it gave Chris the ability to have a look at my lymph nodes, rather than the keyhole surgery which would have been more localised. He could have taken the prostate out, but not been able to do much more.

With the option we chose he was able to take out a whole lot of lymph nodes. I think he took nine out on one side, five on another side. He got a biopsy completed on all of them.

The biopsy showed that there was a trace of cancer in one of the nodes. All the other ones were clear. Obviously he wasn't able to remove all the lymph nodes, only the ones that he could easily have access to. So that is the thing that we've got to constantly now be aware of, and have monitored.

Because I don't have a prostate, my prostate reading has gone to negative 0.5 and it should stay there. But if it looks like it is creeping up, then it is a major alert and a major sign that we didn't capture infected lymph nodes. It means the cancer is starting to come back and we've got to deal with it. Fingers crossed that is not the case and we did get it.

Generally the whole thing was pretty good and I was able to deal with it pretty well. The only real concern I had was when I went in for a computed tomography (CT) scan four days before I saw Chris. That's all about your bones and what's happening to them. I could handle all the other side effects, but if it was my bones that were affected that would be a totally different thing to deal with. Those four days were bloody horrible, but the results were all clear.

I've told all my friends about the whole thing, and I haven't been afraid to give the full details to anyone who asks.

I have told them all to go in and have a medical because that is the benchmark, right? From that point on you have something to measure everything from. So go in and bloody have that done. I have no problem with saying that, because I think the more people know, and do it, the better.

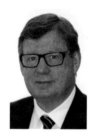

Rob Fisher

Rob Fisher is a barrister who in a 40-year legal career has specialised in resource management, public law and local government law. Rob was the 2010 Barrister of the Year in the New Zealand Law Awards and was made an Officer of the New Zealand Order of Merit in 2011. He is now the company secretary of Auckland City's Watercare. To people outside the legal profession, he's best known as the chairman of the New Zealand Rugby Union from 1997 to 1999, and again in 2002. In 2013 he was diagnosed with prostate cancer.

My cancer was found as part of a regular check-up. I was a partner in a law firm that paid for annual check-ups for partners. Not all partners did them regularly and, in fact, neither did I.

So my first message to people is, if you have an enlightened employer that pays for medical checks, for God's sake, get them done!

When I came to Watercare, they had annual medical checks with the same outfit, and I started going each year.

Over a couple of years my PSA level went up slightly. It had got to 4.7, which is nothing but, because of the trend that had set in, the doctor, Bill Short, said, 'I'm going to send you off for some blood tests and we will have a look at those.' It had gone up to 5.9.

So he sent me off to a urologist. Much to my surprise, I had prostate cancer.

Digital examinations over a period of time had shown nothing. The prostate was not enlarged.

So I had quite a low PSA level, and nothing showing up digitally. It was only my doctor looking at the trend and the small increase that led to further checks.

Then I had a biopsy which came back as a 7 on the Gleason scale. The specialist said, 'If we do nothing you'll probably be fine for up to five years, but thereafter you probably won't be. And at 7, doing nothing in my view is not an option, so really it is radiation or surgery.'

He's a urologist, and I had read that urologists always want to cut and the oncologists want to give you radiation.

But this guy was really good. He said, 'I suggest you get a second opinion,' and he sent me off to a top oncologist. I told him I had pretty well decided on surgery. He said, 'I think that is a good option for you.' I had the surgery and now my PSA level is undetectable.

I was 69 at the time, and that was the factor. I looked at what the doctor had written in a report, and he said, 'despite his age' (the cheeky bugger) 'Rob is very fit and enjoys life to the full, and I think he should deal with this now rather than when he gets older and might not be in such good shape to withstand operations.'

What was interesting, when they got the thing out, is that there was more cancer there than they expected to see given the Gleason score of 7.

After my operation I was back at work within a couple of weeks. Having had four hip replacements I wasn't concerned about surgery, per se. Even with the hip operations I would get back to work after about three weeks, but there was more discomfort with the hip than there was with the prostate surgery.

As I say, a lot of my partners, particularly the younger ones, did not take up what is a very extensive medical which usually takes a good hour and a half. You are on the treadmill all wired up, and all that sort of thing.

A lot of them just didn't do that. That is really silly. A blood test is nothing, and if that detects a trend then you do something a bit more about it before it becomes a serious problem.

EXAMINING THAT GUY

Leigh Hart's been That Guy on Sky's SportsCafe, *a key member of Radio Hauraki's Alternative Cricket Commentary Collective, and appears with Jason Hoyte on Hauraki presenting 'Bhuja!' every weekday from 4pm to 7pm.*

You never forget the first time you have a check-up. I know I certainly won't.

I remember being in my health professional's clinic getting a thorough examination. I recall him gently cupping my testicles in the palm of his hand and asking me to do that little cough thing.

Then he donned a latex surgical glove, asked me to take a deep breath and proceeded to give me a rectal examination.

He seemed to know what he was doing and I am pleased to say that this procedure was nowhere near as bad as I thought it would be. BUT to be honest . . . you don't really expect that from your dentist!

Bowel Cancer
There Is Good News

L et's start with the good news about bowel cancer . . .
Find it early and there's a 99% cure rate.

Find it later and it's still not automatically the end of the world.

Find it at any stage and there's also a very good chance you won't be worrying about a plastic bag attached to your abdomen. There's a process called restorative surgery, where they reattach the ends of the bowel after a portion has been cut out. Only your surgeon will be able to tell the difference.

How do you make sure that if you do get it you're one of the 99% who get better?

If you're only in your 20s and your exercise is getting up from the sofa to get a cold beer from the fridge, or to check on how the ribs are going in the smoker, it'd be a good idea to cut back on the booze and barbecue, and get into any exercise you enjoy as often as you can.

Keeping your weight down, eating a good share of fruit and vegetables, not drinking too much, easing back on fatty meat, salt and sugar will all help. Bowel cancer wards tend not to be full of lean, fit touch footy players.

There's nothing good you can say about bowel cancer, but it is politically correct. It's not sexist. Historically in New Zealand there's little difference between the incidence in men and women, although women are slightly more likely to be affected.

It's not racist. In the past Kiwis of European descent were more likely to have bowel cancer than Maori or Pasifika people. That gap is closing, possibly because of changes in lifestyle and diet.

Whatever your ancestry, if you're heading towards the magic 50 mark, you can really help yourself by tracking down a bit of family history.

Fifty or 60 years ago treatments for cancer, compared to what's available today, were generally so unsuccessful people were scared into silence. There was about as much chance of your grandmother talking about oral sex as there was she'd break into a discussion on exactly what the cancer was that killed her brother.

But there are a couple of questions it'd be very worthwhile to quiz your family about.

One is what close relatives died of. If bowel cancer crops up a couple of times, try to find out what age they were. If they were all over 55 you're at no greater risk than a guy whose family members only die from parachuting accidents.

On the other hand, if your mother, father, brother or sister have had bowel cancer, especially if two or more of them have had it before they turned 50, and you've just had your 50th birthday, don't mess around. Take some action. As they say in the classics, the life you save may be your own. (You can get the exact details of what your risk might be at health.govt.nz/publication/bowel-cancer-information-people-increased-risk-bowel-cancer).

What you can do?

Start with a visit to your doctor. If you don't have one, have a look at the last chapter in this book, 'Picking Your Coach'. If your doctor has concerns, there's a very good chance he or she will recommend a colonoscopy.

A colonoscopy will take a day out of your life, and anywhere from $1600 to $3000 out of your bank balance, if you get it done privately. If the figures make you gasp, the $3000 is very much a worst-case scenario. It is expensive but, in most cases, will be under $2000.

There's a chance you'll get one free from the public health service, but unfortunately waiting lists are lengthy, even for those people with symptoms prompting investigation.

The upside is that it may gift you another 30 or so years of life.

What is a colonoscopy? Basically it's an examination of your colon.

I had a disease called colitis for over 30 years. I also had an older brother who died of bowel cancer before he was 55. Because of those two facts I've had more colonoscopies than Elizabeth Taylor had husbands.

So I can vouch for the fact that while they're not the first thing you'd choose for your next birthday present, they're not painful, just uncomfortable.

You have a colonoscopy in an operating theatre. You're sedated before you go in, at about a 'three or four rum and Cokes' level.

A specialist threads a tiny video camera into your colon through your backside. He or she will be looking for polyps, a small growth on the wall of the colon.

If polyps are found, a section of the polyp is cut off. There is, I swear, no pain, not even a cutting sensation.

The only uncomfortable part is that they may pump a little air into the colon, and you'll feel bloated.

You'll sleep at the hospital for a couple of hours afterwards. As you wake up, you may think for a moment you've accidentally been dropped into the seal colony at Cape Foulwind, because that's what a ward full of sleeping colonoscopy patients farting like horses to get rid of the air sounds and smells a little like.

The next day, after what will almost certainly be a deep sleep at home, you won't even know you've had the procedure.

The biopsies, or small samples of any polyps found, will be examined in a laboratory to see if there are any signs of cancer, or pre-cancerous cells.

Hopefully you'll get the all clear. From here on your doctor will tell you how often, if at all, you need to be checked.

What about if your family tree looks clear of scary cancers? Are there symptoms to look for just in case?

Arend Merrie, Clinical Director of General Surgery at Auckland City Hospital, says there are. Some you can see by looking in your toilet bowl. A change in bowel habit, especially to a looser bowel movement, and even more so if there is mucus or some blood in the motions, needs to be investigated.

So does unexplained weight loss or unexplained anaemia. 'Other symptoms,' says Arend, 'might be vaguer. Bright red bleeding from the bottom end is most likely to be haemorrhoids.'

Whether one or more of the symptoms are worrying you, once again the first step is very straightforward: go to a doctor. The earlier anything is picked up, the better the outcome.

If a decision is made to remove part, or even all, of the bowel, this process has been made easier by massive advances in medical practice and technology over the last 20 years.

What seems a widespread misconception is that a bowel operation means you'll spend the rest of your life with a plastic bag catching your motions (we could say crap, but let's keep it polite).

As I discovered, that's now not the case. Over the last 20 years surgeons have developed what they call a restorative procedure, restoring the bowel's continuity. A layman like you or me might call it reattaching the bowel where they've cut a section out.

'Most people with bowel cancer,' says Arend Merrie, 'wouldn't have the whole colon removed. If you have someone presenting with bowel cancer, the most important thing is to do a good cancer operation. Can you deal with the cancer?

'The second thing then is, can you join things together again? There have been significant advances in that. Nobody likes the concept of a bag. It doesn't matter how permanent or temporary it is, because it's a foreign thing. The reality is that most people who have one say, "It wasn't so bad after all." The concept is often worse than the reality, and that's a very difficult thing to get across.

'Having said that the advances in joining the bowel back together again have been ongoing for 20-odd years.'

What can you expect after your bowel is reconnected? Depending on how much bowel you've had taken out, a lot more visits to the toilet. The more bowel removed (in my case, because I'd had colitis for so many years, I lost the lot), the more time on the toilet.

Why is that? Briefly your digestive system starts with your stomach, which breaks food down. Then things move to the small bowel, where food and drink is digested. What's left moves to the colon (or the first 80 to 100cm of the large bowel) where, if it's working properly, fluid is taken out. The last 15 to 20cm of the large bowel is the rectum, which holds your stools (we could say crap but let's stay polite) until you get rid of them from your anus. Lose too much of your large bowel and what emerges is unlikely to be firm enough to float.

What you don't lose is control so, although you may need a toilet very badly at times, you will be able to hang on until a service station or a public toilet sign appears.

In this country, through the public health system, you will almost certainly receive world-class surgery. Arend Merrie credits improved techniques to pioneers in the 1980s, notably the late Graham Hill, who was the head of surgery at Auckland Hospital, and a professor at Auckland University's School of Medicine.

The standards that Professor Hill and his associates inspired improved the standard of care so much that the recurrence of cancer after operations low in the bowel dropped from 30% to 3% in the 1980s.

Keyhole surgery, as the name implies, reduces the size of the incision needed to get at the colon. Recovery time with keyhole surgery is much less, and getting back to normal life happens much more quickly. Ten or 15 years ago you might have been in hospital for one or two weeks. Today it's more likely to be two to four days.

'We encourage people to get up and around,' says Arend, 'because we know that helps get the gut going, gets breathing working better, and so it reduces the risk of complications.'

No magic bullet has been found for cancers detected at a late stage, but with a combination of surgery, chemotherapy and radiation therapy, even cancers that have spread from the bowel aren't a totally lost cause.

'The imaging in scans has improved. We can use radiotherapy to shrink a tumour to make surgery possible. There have been advances in chemotherapy agents. We now use two or three agents for chemotherapy which improves the outcome. So there have been improvements in all those areas.

'There are fewer patients now,' says Arend, 'to whom we would say, "No, this is not curable." What was once not curable at all can now have a 25% cure rate, which is likely to improve even more.'

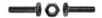

Online, the best place to start looking for more information is the Ministry of Health website at health.govt.nz/your-health/conditions-and-treatments/ diseases-and-illnesses/bowel-cancer.

There you will find, as well as extensive, accurate information, the web addresses of, amongst others, excellent organisations such as the Cancer Society, and Beat Bowel Cancer New Zealand.

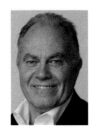

David Vinsen

David Vinsen leads life on the move. For a start, there's his motorbike riding hobby. His business career is a definition of multi-tasking. He's the chief executive of the Imported Motor Vehicle Industry Association (IMVIA), which, as the association has a management agreement with a similar association in Australia, means he's a very frequent trans-Tasman flyer. He and his wife, Mary, are the principals of Quinovic Parnell, a property management company. He chairs the Parnell Community Trust, a preferred service provider for Auckland Council. The trust has 80 staff and runs everything from childhood centres to farmers' markets. There are also Vinsen family property investments in Rarotonga to help supervise. So when, in December 2014, he was diagnosed with bowel cancer, as well as coping on a personal level, there were business ramifications to be considered. What he discovered was heartening. If people are kept informed, a huge fund of goodwill is just waiting to be tapped into.

My advice is that when you go through this process, make preparations and tell people. Don't keep it a secret. Actively solicit support from family, friends and colleagues.

In 2014 I was away overseas in Germany with a motorcycling mate. I happened to notice a bit of blood on the toilet paper. I thought I had haemorrhoids, which I'd never had.

When I got back I had a few things to see my doctor about, and I told him I had this blood on the paper. He said, 'Have you got it now?' And I said, 'No.'

'How long ago was that?'

'About three weeks.' He said to go and get this test done. 'What for?'

'Bowel cancer.' I was expecting him to say haemorrhoids.

He gave me a prescription for tests. I went straight down to Labtests, but when I looked at it, what I had to do was provide three samples over three consecutive days, all to be taken to the laboratory each day. It all seemed too hard, so I chucked it in the cupboard and carried on.

Then, about two weeks later, I got a letter from the Waitemata District Health Board about bowel cancer testing. I thought they were following me up about not doing the test.

Then I read it more carefully, and saw it was something quite separate, part of the pilot scheme they're running for the government. A mass thing for people over a certain age.

Two invitations to participate? The universe is trying to tell me something. So I did both the tests at the same time.

They both came back positive. I went to my doctor, and said, 'What should I do?' Because I had health insurance. He said to go through the public system and see what transpires, and then I could make my call at any stage.

I went through the colonoscopy under the public system. That came back positive. I actually came to during the colonoscopy. I heard the guy say, 'I don't like the look of this one.' He was taking polyps out.

He told me later there was one he didn't like. He thought it was early stage cancer. I liked the sound of 'early stage'. I didn't like the cancer part.

He said I could either go public or private. With Waitemata, if I went public, I'd probably get the same surgeon, the same surgery, and the aftercare would probably be in a room with three other people.

If I went private, I'd have a choice of surgeon and the aftercare would be nicer. The only downside was that if there was an emergency I'd be wheeled back into the public sector.

I took the punt and went private. I was happy with my choice. But I've talked with people who went through the public system who were also very happy with what happened to them.

I had a very positive approach to the whole thing. I decided I was going to write off 2015. I was going to get through it and get well.

I told my board (at the IMVIA) and made no secret about what was going on. I garnered as much support, emotional and practical, as I could.

I read a bit about it, and talked to my surgeon, who was very good. I had the surgery and had the bag.

At first, in hospital, I didn't want to see my stoma (the opening in the abdomen that allows waste to pass into a bag). The first time I looked at it was when I was in the shower, and I looked at the reflection in a mirror. Then I had a proper look at it. I had very good nursing staff who helped me and I got used to dealing with it.

I had no real problems. There were just some inconveniences dealing with it.

Shortly before my surgery I'd gone to a mate's 60th in Christchurch on my bike. I flew back. Four months later I flew down, picked up the bike, and started riding home. I was in my riding gear, having a sleep on the ferry, when I woke and found I'd messed myself inside my riding gear. People on the ferry were wonderful. They took me into a staff shower, got me plastic bags, wipes, just brilliant.

So I cleaned myself up, stayed at a mate's place in Waikanae and rode to Bulls. By the time I got there it happened again. I cleaned myself up in a café toilet in Bulls, put my last bag on, and by the time I got up to Foxton, it had happened again. The way I was crouched up on the bike was causing it.

That was the only time I had a problem. I had a really good stoma nurse who talked me through it. It wasn't a big deal.

I've got two elderly friends who have had the same procedure. They talked with friends and decided they'd keep their bags, rather than go through the reversal surgery. They're quite comfortable managing the bag.

I had my bag taken off in June 2015. The real process for me had been quite smooth, always looking to see a positive outcome at the end.

I hadn't fully understood what the reconnection meant. I hadn't realised that in taking away 850mm of my lower bowel, that the lower bowel's function was to remove water and store waste. The water in a normal full-sized bowel gets taken out. You've lost that ability to remove water and compact the contents.

At first there was a daily cycle where I would feel bloated and constipated, then I'd start to go to the toilet, then almost normal, then diarrhoea and sometimes quite painful wind.

The surgeon said it could be two years before it came right. I started to take small doses of the pills travellers use for dysentery overseas, and I have Metamucil, a soluble fibre drink, every morning. Six months into it I began to feel really good.

Obviously I wish I'd rather not have had it at all. But I'm very pleased with how it's been treated.

I've been running the IMVIA for 13 years, but I also have a

portfolio career, so I had a whole variety of things that I had to put on hold, and make arrangements for.

When I told my IMVIA board about it, they said, 'Right, you do whatever you have to do to get better.' Early on it was announced in trade magazines *Autotalk* and *Autofile* that I was taking sick leave, so everybody knew. There was no suggestion of covering up. Not bleating about it, just stating the facts. 'Here's the deal. I might need your help.'

Everybody, in every case, stuck their hand up to help. In the property business franchise that Mary and I have, the franchise chairman Ross Davey, who understood what I was going through, flew up from Wellington to tell us the franchise would provide any assistance necessary to our business. Fortunately we have really good staff, so we didn't actually need it.

But that was completely indicative of how people will assist you if you're straight up and tell them, even ask for help.

What happens is that when people hear about your health issue they feel impotent. They empathise, they sympathise, but they don't know what to do to help.

If you say to them, 'Look, there's some practical stuff you can do to help, would you mind doing this? Would you mind looking after Australia for me for six months, because I can't travel?' They say, 'Absolutely, no problem.' Think about the practical things you need to be able to carry on.

I couldn't drive for a while, but when I started getting back on track, when a lot of my work consisted of meetings, all my colleagues were quite happy to truck out from the city to West Harbour, and we'd have meetings at home, or they'd pick me up and we'd go to a local café, and have the meeting there. It was really great.

The other thing I was told, which I now subscribe to, is rest. Don't feel awkward about needing lots of rest. Your body needs lots of sleep to heal and recover. Listen to your body. If you need a sleep in the afternoon, don't fight it.

Also, take into account the effect on your partner and family. You tend to focus on yourself. I was lucky, because I had a colleague, and she told me, 'Make sure you look after your wife.' She'd had cancer some years ago, and the effect on her husband was devastating. He struggled to cope with it. She said, 'Make sure you look after each other.' In our case, Mary had some professional counselling. She was trying to be strong for me, bottling it all up, and that had a deleterious effect on her.

A friend in the motor industry said to me, 'At our age we have to be kind to ourselves, and we have to be kind to each other.' Take the hard edge of aggression off what we do. There's no reason why we can't be kinder to ourselves, and nicer to other people.

So my advice is, get tested, and if you happen to get caught, don't be backward in putting your hand up, and asking people for help. In my experience, they'll respond positively.

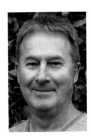

Bill Molloy

Bill Molloy is a true southern man. He was born and bred in Southland, training to be a mine surveyor. In 1985 he played on the wing for Southland against the touring England rugby side. Twenty years ago, his work took him to the West Coast, where he's lived ever since. After three years of treatment for Paget's disease of the anus, he was diagnosed with bowel cancer just before Christmas in 2009.

My cancer experience started in mid-2005. It began with a nasty rash, which steroid cream from the doctor only made worse.

So, after a few weeks of that, I ended up having a biopsy taken, and was diagnosed with Paget's disease of the anus. I was told it's quite rare and affects different people in different ways. Women can get it in the breast, and you can get it in the bones as well.

For me it was a non-invasive form of skin cancer. It required me to have an operation to remove the area that was affected. But with Paget's disease it is normally a secondary form of cancer, often associated with bowel cancer.

So, I ended up having to go to Christchurch to see a specialist, Professor Frank Frizelle, to get the operation for Paget's disease done.

I was quite fortunate, as he is one of the top bowel cancer authorities in New Zealand. After the operation, he started me on a course of checks to see whether I had bowel cancer.

There were all sorts of things that went on after that, examinations, blood tests, CT scans; all sorts of things to try to determine whether there was a primary source of cancer. But the tests didn't show anything.

Then I went on to regular check-ups with Frank. This went on for another two or three years.

It was during my second colonoscopy, about four years after I had my initial surgery for the Paget's disease, that Frank found a growth in my rectum, which proved to be bowel cancer. That was in December 2009.

It wasn't a very good Christmas present. Frank advised me that I needed to have an operation, but before that I also needed courses of chemotherapy and radiation treatment. That started in February 2010, and I had six weeks of chemotherapy and radiation treatment simultaneously.

The chemotherapy was continuous for six weeks. I had a PICC line (a catheter or small tube) inserted into my arm, and that went up to the top of my heart, and there was a little automatic pump that I used to wear in a bum bag that was connected to that. So that was continuously dripping chemotherapy drugs into my system, 24/7 for six weeks.

I had to stay in Christchurch for six weeks. To be honest, I thought it was going to be a lot more drastic than it was. I didn't really know, but I thought I was going to lose all my hair, like you hear all these stories, how you get really sick.

The chemo drug they put me on was called 5-Fluorouracil (5FU) and I found it quite a tolerable sort of a drug. After a couple of weeks the only real symptom I had was that I got very tired. I didn't lose any of my hair or anything like that. I just lost some energy.

For the radiation treatment I had to stay in Christchurch, because it was at the Christchurch hospital. That was five days a week, Monday to Friday. So I had a timetable right through for the whole six weeks with times I had to go and what machine I had to go on.

We were quite fortunate, because we owned an apartment in Christchurch at the time, basically a holiday home. Our son went to school there, and then to university, and our daughter was doing a beauty therapy course. So we had a base in Christchurch.

Once the six weeks was up, I had a two-week rest prior to the operation, although I went back to work for about a week of that.

I'd worked for Solid Energy and its predecessors for so long, I had clocked up 37 years with them, so I had quite a lot of sick leave owing. They let me take my sick leave and I ended up having about, in total, probably three or four months off work.

Two weeks after the radiation and chemo I had the operation in Christchurch at St Georges Hospital. Through Solid Energy I had medical insurance, which was a blessing. That enabled me to go private for my operation.

I don't think any private hospitals in Christchurch at that time had any radiation treatment facilities. It was all done at Christchurch Hospital. I just can't thank the radiation nurses and staff enough, they were just absolutely fantastic through that whole process.

With the operation I was told right from the start that I would have a permanent colostomy bag because the cancer was so low down — it was in my rectum; it wasn't actually in the colon.

Well, they had to take out the whole of the rectum. The technical term is an abdominoperineal resection. They took out the rectum, which included the anus and about 20 centimetres of the lower part of the colon. Basically they sewed up my bum.

The operation was a lot bigger than I thought it would be. It lasted between three and four hours, and affected me a lot more than I expected.

I had an allergic reaction to one of the anti-nausea drugs. Fortunately one of the nurses realised what was going on and they put me on other drugs, and after six days in hospital I was fine.

But once I left and went back to the apartment, I was very ill, throwing up for Africa. For about a fortnight I pretty much lived on Powerade. It was probably six months before I felt I was really over the operation.

As to having to have a colostomy bag for the rest of my life, at first I thought to myself, 'That is going to be horrible. Why me?' I started feeling sorry for myself. But every time I'd do that I would wake myself up and say, 'Bill, you're okay, you're alive.' There was only one other option, being dead, and I didn't want to take that one!

I had a stoma (an opening) just across from my bellybutton, and I now have a bag attached there all the time.

When I was in Christchurch recovering, a nurse would come around and check me. They taught me about life with a colostomy bag, how to care for it, how to care for the stoma and the skin around it. I got a lot of good advice from Nurse Maude in Christchurch, and subsequently the stoma nurse here in Greymouth gave me information.

It doesn't take long at all to get used to. One catastrophe I do remember. At night I woke up and things weren't too good. It had come apart. And that's the worst experience I've had. That's not too bad, one experience like that over six years.

There are not many things that I don't do that I used to be able to do before. I play golf regularly. I still travel. My wife and I have been overseas on a couple of big holidays since I've had my bag.

It hasn't really stopped me doing too much. I don't strip off when it's hot in the summertime and go swimming or anything like that any more. I am quite conscious of the fact that I have a bag and I don't advertise the fact that I've got it.

I'm still working. For many years I was in the technical services department at the Spring Creek mine for Solid Energy. A few years after my operation a job came up at a local civil construction company, and I've been working for them for three years, mostly in contract administration.

I have regular checks still. It started out every three months and now it's a yearly check.

I've also gone back to make sure that I get things checked if I'm not happy about something, that's for sure. For me, not knowing is the worst thing because you tend to think the worst. But, so far, so good.

BILLY T'S FAVOURITE

Our most popular comedian, the late, great Billy T James, picked his six favourite jokes for a story in a magazine I was editing in 1985. Here's the one he said was his favourite.

A big container ship is heading north from New Zealand to the Pacific Islands. The crew sight what's obviously the wreckage of a yacht, and the huge ship is slowed to a halt. Among the debris is a survivor. The container ship's skipper, a Kiwi, calls down: 'What nationality are you?' The survivor calls back: 'I'm English.' The skipper says: 'What's the worst maritime disaster there's ever been?'

'That'd be the *Titanic*.'

'Haul him up.'

The ship continues for another few hundred metres and there is another survivor of the wreck. 'What nationality are you?'

'American.'

'What's the worst maritime disaster there's ever been?'

'The *Titanic*.'

'How many people perished?'

'About 1100.'

'Haul him up.'

A few hundred metres more and they find a third survivor, 'What nationality?'

'Australian.'

'What's the worst maritime disaster?'

'The *Titanic*.'

'How many perished?'

'About 1100.'

Pause. 'Name them.'

Your Heart
The Magic Machine in Your Chest

Your heart is an amazing machine. Every day it pumps about 7200 litres of blood around your body. By the end of a month that means it has pumped enough blood to fill an Olympic sized swimming pool.

Your heart is a muscle. Bulging biceps and six-pack abs look great, but really the heart is the most important muscle in your body. Only the size of your fist, it sits in your chest between your lungs, usually a little to the left side.

When your heart's healthy it's not only strong, but beautifully designed.

It's divided into four chambers, linked by valves that open and shut like gates, to keep the blood flowing like a one-way traffic system.

In very basic terms, blood that's been around your body and is low in oxygen flows into the two chambers on the right side of your heart. The heart pumps it through your lungs, where it becomes oxygen rich. The oxygen-rich blood comes back to the two chambers on the left side of your heart, and is then pumped around your body.

A heart attack happens when an artery on the surface of your heart (one which feeds the heart muscle with the oxygen-rich blood) blocks, usually suddenly, and so the blood supply to your heart is stopped.

With no disrespect to the talented health experts who patch your heart up if it fails, nobody can keep it healthy as well as you can.

We'll get to what the experts do later in the chapter, but right now there are some very straightforward ways to make sure you'll never be staring at the roof of an ambulance wondering how the hell that indigestion that had been bugging you for a few days had suddenly become a full-blown heart attack.

Not smoking is one guaranteed way to reduce the risk of a heart problem. In the chapter 'Stubbing Out the Habit' there are suggestions to help you break the treacherous addiction.

Nic Gill, the All Blacks' fitness trainer, in the chapter 'Finding Your Fun', offers tips on exercise and diet to help your general fitness, which is a vital part of heart care. Lee-Anne Wann, a nutritionist who advises, amongst others, the Warriors, gives advice on healthy eating in 'Great Food: That Doesn't Taste Like Crap'. We've also included chapters on places to go in New Zealand, and things to do, read and see that help reduce stress, another problem for the health of your heart.

(In passing, and I am not making this up, when the All Blacks lose at a World Cup, numbers for heart failure go through the roof. A 2014 report by two Christchurch doctors shows that for some fans, if the All Blacks don't win, it can literally be heart breaking. When we lost the semi-final in 1999, admissions to New Zealand hospitals for heart attacks went up 33%. When the All Blacks lost in Sydney in 2003, heart attacks went up 60%.)

Keeping yourself fit, and your cholesterol level down, does you a double favour. 'Everything you do for yourself that is beneficial to reducing your risk of having a heart attack,' says cardiologist Gerry Devlin, Medical Director of the New Zealand Heart Foundation, 'is also reducing your risk of having a stroke. It's an important message, because we don't always put those two things together. Stopping smoking and making sure your blood pressure and blood sugar are normal also reduce your chances of developing heart disease and stroke.'

The best way to describe a stroke, he says, is calling it a 'brain attack', because the causes are exactly the same as a heart attack.

'A stroke usually occurs when you have the blood supply completely interrupted to the brain. It is the same mechanism in the arteries or the blood supply as in a heart attack. And then you have a brain attack, or a stroke. You can also have bleeds in the brain that can cause strokes, but the bleed is less common. It is usually the stoppage of the blood to the brain.'

If your heart starts to flag, the warning signs can be very subtle.

The movies' version, the grabbing of the chest, the gasping, the eye rolling, the (if you're Marlon Brando in *The Godfather*) crashing into the garden and scaring the crap out of your grandson, might happen, but it's unlikely.

Sometimes the symptoms are so unremarkable it's almost a case of attack by tedium.

'More often than not,' says Gerry Devlin, 'you may just feel a bit of discomfort, or feel uncomfortable in the chest, jaw, or arm.

'I try to use the word "discomfort" when I talk to medical students and patients, because the classic Hollywood tightness, really bad tightness where you feel your chest has been crushed, yes it happens, but it is less likely.

'What I ask patients is, "Are you getting discomfort in your chest when you do things? When you're under stress. Say, watching a rugby match." The All Blacks in 2015 at the World Cup, for example, came close a couple of times! So it can be emotional or physical stress.

'If you notice when you are walking up a hill, or doing the lawns, that your chest feels a bit uncomfortable, your throat feels a bit uncomfortable, we would say don't ignore that, that is something that you should go and talk to your health professional about.

'A lot of people who have heart attacks often have those symptoms building up for a few weeks beforehand.'

You can check the excellent website, heartfoundation.org.nz, for more details on what to look for in case you're starting to have a heart attack.

But if you're not too great on the world web net thing, here are the signs to look out for.

The discomfort Gerry Devlin talks about may come and go. It may be in one, or both, arms but is more likely to be in the left arm. It can be in your neck, your jaw, your stomach, or your abdomen.

What does it actually feel like? It can be squeezing, pressing, tightness, feeling full, or actual pain. You might also find yourself sweating, being faint or dizzy, feeling that you want to throw up, actually vomiting, or being short of breath.

'The message for middle-aged blokes,' says Gerry Devlin, 'is if you're getting discomfort in your chest, arm or throat when you are doing things, if you believe something is not quite right, and you are feeling things are harder for you to do, then don't ignore it. Go and see a doctor.

'The fact is statistics show that we never get to see 50% of people who have a heart attack until after it happens.'

Being an active, non-smoking, healthy eater remains the best armour to wear to ward off a heart attack.

But even if you jog six days a week, and are so health-food conscious you feel a little nauseated just at the sight of a fried chicken ad on TV, there are some medical precautions that are worth taking.

Experts in the heart field recommend you start getting your heart checked by your doctor from the age of 45.

You should get tested about 10 years younger if you're Maori, because statistics show Maori men have a slightly higher risk of heart problems.

If there's a family history of heart disease, that should set off what Gerry Devlin calls 'an amber warning light' and lead you to having tests done earlier. If your dad died of a heart attack in his early 60s, beat the problem to the punch and get yourself checked out.

If you go to your GP, what's likely to be involved?

Nothing that's stressful. He or she will take your blood pressure. Blood tests will be ordered to check out your cholesterol levels and see what your blood sugar levels are. Results from the blood tests can provide an early-warning sign.

Your doctor, or a specialist, if it's decided you should see one, may run more tests.

A common test is an electrocardiogram or ECG in which electrodes are attached to your chest, you lie down for about 10 minutes, and what your heart is doing is monitored. The electrodes are attached by a paste. There's no pain involved. The worst that can happen is if you're a very manly man with a lot of chest hair, some of it may be shaved off.

Another test is taken while you're on a treadmill, wired up in the same way as you would be for an ECG. There will also be a blood pressure monitor wound around your arm. Depending on your level of fitness you'll be asked to walk or jog, while measurements are recorded.

The inconvenience is genuinely minor. The rewards in spotting a problem early, when it can be solved, are huge. More good news is the fact it's never been easier in New Zealand to get access to a cardiologist, to have thorough tests done.

Hopefully you'll be fine. If you're not, you've come to the right country to get well.

For a start, the treatment will be timely. Twenty-five years ago, says Gerry Devlin, you waited 18 months for a heart bypass operation in the public health system. Now nobody waits more than three months. The result is that a graph of the number of deaths from heart disease over the last 40 years shows a line that points steeply downwards.

Why has there been such a dramatic improvement? Says Gerry: 'It is probably about 50% due to the medicines and 50% due to better surgery, with more access to surgery and stents.'

What exactly is involved in having bypass surgery, and what are stents?

Stents are very small metal mesh tubes that cardiologists put inside the arteries of the heart where there's a blockage or a narrowing. What's called a balloon treatment opens the artery, and a stent is used to keep the artery open. It will usually stay in the artery for the rest of your life. Special coating on today's stents mean very few narrow with time, but in around 5 to 10% of cases after some years there may be a need to put another stent inside the old stent, or to have a bypass operation.

What's a bypass? Exactly what it says. Blood is being blocked in an artery going into your heart. If a stent won't open it, the alternative is to get the blood around the blockage.

A surgeon takes a small section of blood vessel, usually from your leg, arm or chest. One end is attached at the top of the blockage, the other at the bottom. The blood flows past the danger area, the same way a bypass on the road diverts traffic around an accident or roadworks.

Angina is something that occurs when an artery is narrowing, but is not actually closed. Your heart is not getting enough blood and, as it is a muscle, albeit an amazingly sophisticated and vital muscle, it starts to hurt.

Gerry Devlin says the first signs of angina will usually occur when your heart is put under pressure. 'It may feel okay when you're sitting down, doing nothing, but if you're walking in a cold wind, or up a hill, and you need a little more blood, the discomfort or pain you will feel is the heart muscle.

'You're not having a heart attack if you have angina, but angina can lead on to a heart attack. If this muscle is not getting enough blood to it, and it stays like that for a long time, then the muscle starts to die and that is when you get a heart attack. The pain of a heart attack, compared to angina, tends to be a bit more severe.'

If you do suffer a heart attack, the days of someone who had a heart operation, staying for a long time in hospital, and coming home to be treated like an invalid, have gone.

'We don't wrap people up in a blanket and put them in a car to go home,' says Gerry Devlin. 'Years ago, you had a heart attack and you were put in bed for four to six weeks and that was probably it. Now we do what we can to keep people well, and to keep them doing what they want to do.

'Life expectancy is going up and up all the time, at a phenomenal rate. So we have the challenge of helping people with heart disease live life to the full. That is what it is about now.'

Cardiac arrest

When Warriors and former All Blacks doctor John Mayhew almost died in April 2016, it was the first time many of us were made aware that a heart attack and cardiac arrest are different things.

John had just finished a CrossFit gym session when he collapsed. He had suffered cardiac arrest, caused by a virus that had damaged his heart. Not a heart attack.

He says, 'A cardiac arrest happens when your heart stops pumping blood around your body.' A heart attack is when part of the heart muscle dies because of blockage in one of the coronary arteries, so a lot of heart attacks can cause cardiac arrests. The most common cause of a cardiac arrest is a life-threatening abnormal heart rhythm called ventricular fibrillation (VF), which is most frequently caused by heart attacks.

A cardiac arrest is an emergency. Someone who is having a cardiac arrest will suddenly lose consciousness and will stop breathing or stop breathing normally. Unless immediately treated by cardiopulmonary resuscitation or CPR (which involves pressure on the chest, and breathing into the collapsed person's mouth) this always leads to death within minutes.

VF can sometimes be corrected by giving an electric shock through the chest wall using a device called a defibrillator. For a good description of what defibrillators are, go to this section of the British Heart Foundation website, bhf.org.uk/heart-health/how-to-save-a-life/defibrillators.

Using a defibrillator can be done in the ambulance, or at hospital, or it can be done by a member of the public at the scene of a cardiac arrest if there is a community defibrillator nearby. For every minute without CPR or defibrillation, a patient's chance of survival falls by 10 to 15%.

You can survive and recover from a cardiac arrest, as John Mayhew did, if you get the right treatment quickly.

An off-duty police officer was at the gym at the time he collapsed, and started cardiac massage while someone got a defibrillator.

'I was successfully resuscitated,' says John, 'and after a three-day spell in intensive care in hospital on a ventilator I woke up with no neurological problems.'

So survival from cardiac arrest is possible, but it does depend on, for a start, how many Kiwis know how to do CPR. To learn how to apply CPR the best place to start is with St John. If you go to stjohn.org.nz, you can find where and when to attend classes.

Sadly, CPR alone usually won't save someone suffering cardiac arrest. Recent New Zealand statistics show that while 64% of patients with a cardiac arrest in the community had bystander CPR performed, only 4% of patients were defibrillated using a public access defibrillator called an automated external defibrillator (AED). New Zealand's low rate of public access to defibrillators remains an issue.

Without getting too technical, an AED is a portable medical device that can automatically assess a patient's heart rhythm. It judges whether defibrillation is needed and, if required, administers an electric shock through the chest wall to the heart.

When an AED is used within three minutes of cardiac arrest 75% of patients survive. To learn more about AEDs, a great place to check out is a company, endorsed by John Mayhew, called Heart Saver. Their website is heartsaver.co.nz.

The moral is really very simple. Every day five Kiwis suffer cardiac arrest. More access to AEDs, in gyms, shops, offices, factories, schools, and other public places, means more New Zealanders will live.

The New Zealand Heart Foundation's website is heartfoundation.org.nz.

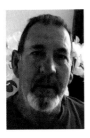

Darryl Potier

Darryl Potier has worked in the building trade all his life. As a teenage league player, he took an apprenticeship as a builder and, at 68, he has just retired from Placemakers, where he worked as an advisor to builders. He's active, a busy home handyman and, with his wife Lenore, a keen dancer at the Whangaparaoa Rock 'n' roll Club. In 2015 he had a heart attack.

We were coming back from Whangamata and when we got back to our home at Arkles Bay I thought I had indigestion.

I didn't feel right, to be fair. The pain didn't dissipate. I was taking Gaviscon, which didn't really help the problem. I said to Lenore, 'I think it's about time to go to the doctor and find out what's going on.'

I'd never had any heart problems before. Nothing had ever shown up. I had already had one of those tests where you go on the exercise bike. I'd had all that done probably six months prior to this happening. I was as good as gold.

So I never ever thought I had anything else but indigestion. My comment to my doctor was I felt it was indigestion that wouldn't go away. Did he know what it was? He gave me an ECG right there at the doctor's surgery and told me we needed to do some blood tests.

But it wasn't until a week later when I was told that the proteins in my blood were elevated (during a heart attack, heart muscle cells die and release proteins into the bloodstream that are picked up in a blood test) that I found out I'd actually had a heart attack. Without knowing.

I was rung up at 9pm on a Wednesday by the doctor and told that I needed to go to hospital. I said to him, 'I'll just get in my car, mate, and I'll roll up there.' He said, 'Well, you can't do that because we're getting you in an ambulance and you're going to go straight to Accident and Emergency.'

I've got a GP who has handled my case over the years since we've been in Whangaparaoa. A few years before I was treated for prostate cancer, so he was keeping an eye on that.

Also, I suffered from high blood pressure, which is part of the concern about having a heart attack or a stroke. I was always on medication for my blood pressure.

The thing is, in the case of a lot of guys, it's hard to tell when you've had a heart attack. Most of us don't admit to the fact that there is something wrong with us but, talking with other men in hospital who had heart attacks, if you've got a sore neck, or jaw, or it's sore in your shoulder, you know that there is something not quite right. You just don't realise it's a heart attack.

They took me to North Shore Hospital, to Accident and Emergency, where they take you in without having to sit around. They were prepared for me. They put me in a room, lay me down, and put me on all the monitors.

It would have been a good day and a half later that the house surgeon came in. Then it was sort of a wait and see game. Eventually I got the angiogram done and that showed blockages had caused my arteries to be from 50 to 80% closed. From then on, it was basically 'there are not many choices, you have to have the bypass, there is nothing else we can do for you'.

In an angiogram, they inject dye into your heart arteries. First they give you a mild sedative just to keep you calm. I have to say, for me, I didn't find it invasive at all. I've talked to other people and they've said they didn't really like it, but I didn't find that to be the way I felt about it. I didn't even know I'd had it done! The guy said, 'I'll give you a little cut,' and the next minute when they pulled it out they just said, 'There is nothing we can repair for you with a stent, we need to look at a bypass operation.'

So then I was waiting in North Shore Hospital for three weeks and moving on to Auckland from there.

There's a huge number of people who've got the same issues that I had. There are probably eight heart operations a day in Auckland

Hospital. They have got great surgeons — well, I would say, the best surgeons in the world — up there.

At Auckland Hospital I had a quadruple bypass. They take veins from your legs and replace the blocked arteries in your heart. If you think about it, it is incredible for someone to be able to take your heart out of your chest and bypass blockages.

They do tell you — and they don't beat around the bush — what could happen inside that theatre. You know when you have that final jab in your arm that either you're going to come out of this or there isn't going to be much else to worry about.

But they're professional people and it is like anybody who has an operation, we leave all the care and attention to them.

From the time I had the operation to the time I went home was only about seven days. So it was a very, very quick turnover.

There is a procedure to the recovery. Basically rest. I was told not to lift anything too heavy, nothing above your chest because obviously the operation is about cutting your ribcage open and refastening it with wire and all of that takes ages to mend together.

There was a case I was told about where a guy went home and, after three weeks, he decided he felt pretty good and he went out and started chopping firewood. They tell you not to do that sort of thing.

But they do say to get out there and walk, which is what I did. You build it up. The first time I ever walked, I'd be lucky if I could walk for five minutes without really puffing. Then after about a week or maybe two weeks I was doing 20 minutes. Probably puffing, but not as badly.

Then, as time went by, before I went back to work I was walking 30 or maybe 40 minutes twice a day. Not so much out on the roads, I was just doing it around the house and rolling along. A couple of times I went on the road but, to me, it just felt a little bit better at home. I didn't really want to be out there in the middle of the road.

I'm lucky enough to have a house that takes a couple of minutes to walk around and on a flat, level surface. I was back at work in July. So from April until the end of June I was convalescing. Altogether it was about two months off work after coming home from hospital.

During that recovery time there was no pain. None at all. The interesting thing is, when you are in hospital you have all the people around you, so you feel very confident that if you have another heart attack or if something happens there are people there who are going to look after you. Initially, when I went home, I had Lenore there, but I felt quite alone. I kept thinking, 'What if I have a heart attack?' and was a little bit frightened about what was going to happen. I think the first couple of nights I was a bit panicky. But as the weeks went by it got much better. When you head home from hospital they give you phone numbers to call if anything happens, so you do have a backup.

The skills shown and the information they give you in hospital are wonderful. I just felt that the doctors and nurses were fantastic.

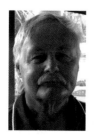

Walter Gill

Walter Gill is a New Zealand discus champion from 1975, who has made his living since the 1970s in a highly successful concrete company with his great friend, round-the-world yachtsman Simon Gundry. Their company motto reflects their quirky sense of humour: 'We may be rough, but at least we're slow.' He is married to Nerida, also a former athlete. Their son, Jacko Gill, has set several world age-group records with the shot. Now 65, when Walter was 62 he suffered a heart attack.

I was a typical sort of guy when I was young. I ate heaps at night-time and if there was any dessert left that would become a late feed. So, consequently, I was used to lying in bed and thinking, 'Jesus, I'm tight in the stomach' and feeling rumbling and what-not. That's how it put me off the scent a bit of what was happening to me.

There were times when I would wake up at night and I would have this burning pain right up the middle of my chest. I'd sit on the side of the bed and maybe have a bit of Mylanta. I used to have a little jar of Mylanta stuck in my drawer there, and I'd have a swig on that and I'd sit there for five minutes and it was gone.

I thought, 'Oh I've fixed that.' And that is what I hadn't done. You never fix it. Then I would lie back and I'd go to sleep and wake up in the morning feeling fine.

I've always been terrified of going to doctors. Dentists don't bother me, pain is nothing, but I've always dreaded being told you've got something bad. It's a fear I've always had. So I didn't get checked by a doctor. I guess there are a lot of people like that, and a lot of braver ones too.

One day I was at work and this pain came on. This time it wasn't in the middle of the night, it was about three in the afternoon. I thought, 'Oh Jeez.' The pain was unbelievable. Just a strange pain. I still thought it was my stomach and indigestion and it felt like it was searing through, as if it had burnt through something, like gone through to somewhere where it shouldn't. I never for a minute thought I was having a heart attack. Not for a minute.

I tried the old method that worked for everything — I'll have a sandwich. And I thought, 'That'll settle my tummy down.' I thought it was just stomach acid so I'll shove something in there. I remember wandering up the hill to my truck and I was taking it slow, and I never realised how dangerous that was.

I sat in my truck and had the sandwich and, when I got out, my stomach went berserk. It was loud rumblings. Just the noise and things, it was just like an absolute fit. Anyway, that eventually died down. I sat in my truck for a bit. I thought, 'I'll sit, the boys are still working.' And eventually it got so sore, I thought, 'No, that is definitely stomach acid that's gone through; it's burned through to somewhere it shouldn't be.'

I was beginning to think, 'I'm in strife here.' I went home and I was still then thinking that it would settle down as it always had. I sat in the lounge for a bit. Then I thought, 'I'll have a shower, that'll freshen me up.' I had all these really good methods! So I started to have a shower and I couldn't finish it. I couldn't finish the shower. It was like . . . wow, the pain was just too much.

I got out and there was nobody home. By this time it was probably five o'clock. They say there is a critical two-hour period that you are meant to get treatment for your heart before it starts doing damage to the heart itself.

Of course, I knew none of this. By then the two hours were already up. Lo and behold, Nerry came home and I said, 'I've really got a bad pain here, I am really sore, I think it's my reflux.'

It was then I made the decision: 'Can you take me to the hospital?' That was pretty big for me. I hated hospitals, I had a fear of just going there. I'd had several incidents previously in my life where I'd been in hospitals and I know they are there to help you, but I just hated being there. To be honest, I was terrified. It was something that really scared me.

Anyway, Nerry drove me to the hospital. We never rang for an ambulance, which was a mistake. You can get help instantly, when they come. But we drove to North Shore Hospital and as soon as I said, 'Look, I've got this searing pain up here,' it was straight in.

Anyone who ever moans about the health service gets an earful from me. I tell you, it was straight in, straight on the bed, they quickly took a blood test and within minutes they said, 'Mr Gill, you are having a heart attack.'

They asked how much I weighed, which was 125kg, which makes you sound like a bit of a hog. But I wasn't really a beach ball. If you'd taken 10kg off I would have been very lean for me.

They also picked up that I had diabetes, and I have to admit I wasn't taking care of that the way I should have been. Apparently that can bring on a heart attack too.

At that time of the night the cardiac department had closed at North Shore for any operations, but Auckland was still functioning, so I was shoved in the back of the ambulance. This all happened in minutes, probably only 15 minutes. I was shoved in there and two ladies got in with me. I didn't fully realise it at the time, but they were St John's people there to resuscitate me if something went wrong.

Nerry hadn't realised the gravity of the situation either. She said, 'I'll go home and get you some clean clothes and stuff,' because I was still in my work gear. Now she says, 'What the hell was I thinking?'

I can remember backing up to the doors to Auckland Hospital. I was wheeled out the back quickly. About three sets of doors opened and then there were bright lights above me.

I was in the operating theatre and they said, 'Hello, Mr Gill, in a little bit of trouble are we?' I said, 'Jesus, yes!' The surgeon said, 'We won't be a minute.' In those few minutes the whole operating staff was assembled.

So immediately they started work. They put dye in and they found the blockage. The surgeon showed me on the screen what it was and what they were going to do. I probably didn't hear that much of it.

I'd never really left myself in somebody else's hands before. I didn't ask people for favours in my life. I'd been one of those kinds of people. But, at that point, I was well aware that I was probably finished if these people didn't help me.

They put in a stent. They put it through your wrist now. It used to be through the groin. But they did it up through the wrist and you can look up at the screen. I opted not to. You can see it going through your system. It gets to where the blockage is and then they inflate it, or something like that. I'm not quite sure how it works.

You're awake through it all. That pleased me because I've got a great fear of being put to sleep. I really don't like the anaesthetic. I can't recall it, but they must have given me something to help me relax. I don't remember there being any pain.

After it was finished the surgeon showed me the picture of what they'd done. He said the artery had been 83% closed.

He said there are two major arteries going into the heart. He called one the Widow Maker. Those are the guys that you see walking along the street, and bang, they're gone. That would be a blockage in the Widow Maker.

He told me mine was in the other one, where you are still getting a flow through. But, in saying that, you wouldn't last long if that shut down 100%. Mine was only 17% open, hence the pain.

Anyway, I was put in a room then and they came in every hour and checked on me. I think all the readings must have been good. It was almost instantly better; the pain had all gone by then. It was instant really, once that blockage was gone and the blood was flowing through again. From there I think I was two days in Auckland Hospital and then transferred back to North Shore.

When the doctors come around, they do all these tests on you. A guy gave me an ultrasound to see how much of the heart had died, because I was well outside that time when it should still be safe. And none of it had. Unbelievable! I was really lucky.

He said it was the best heart he'd seen in there for months. I think it helped that I've never smoked in my life. For any young guy, that is critical.

I used to hang out with the tough guys, who all smoked. I was just starting to throw discus at the time and I think they accepted that I wasn't doing what they all did, because they said, 'Oh, you're a sportsman.' It was kind of a blessing throwing the discus, in many ways. It got me out of poverty, growing up in the worst house in the worst street. While I was never international class, it saved me. You've got no idea.

The guy I saw at the end, when I was getting the final clearance, whose name was Dr Hart, believe it or not, said, 'I wouldn't expect to see you before 18 years.' I don't know why he chose 18 years, maybe he knows something I don't! He said it looked good and just carry on with your life as normal. I'm back doing physical work with the boys.

The diabetes could bring something on again, with my heart. Since then my doctor has made an extreme effort to make sure that is under control. And I have too.

10 Places
to Make You Feel Good About Being a Kiwi

Jim Eagles is the former travel editor of the New Zealand Herald. *He's circled the globe, seen the wonders of the world we've heard of, and many we haven't. He's always had a special spot in his heart for New Zealand. Here are the places that will be good for your soul.*

Cape Reinga. To begin at the beginning (or the end), Cape Reinga, Te Rerenga Wairua, the leaping-off place of spirits, is a stunning spot in every way. To Maori it was, as the name says, the spot from which the souls of the dead departed for Hawaiki, and you can still see the pohutukawa root from which they clung before leaving Aotearoa for the last time. It's certainly a place with a special, almost spiritual, atmosphere. If you choose not to believe that this is caused by the passage of souls, you might prefer it to be due to the mighty Pacific Ocean and the Tasman Sea crashing into each other just off the end

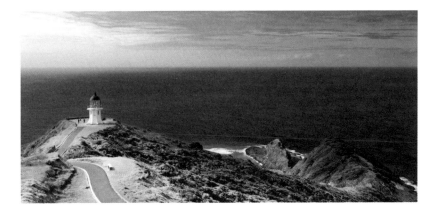

of the cape, creating a line of massive waves and filling the air with the sort of electricity you feel in great storms. If the views from this extraordinary place aren't inspiration enough, Cape Reinga is also the starting point of Te Araroa, the long pathway, our national walkway, which weaves its way down the length of the country to Bluff. The first section of the walkway, from the cape to Ninety Mile Beach, showcases some of the finest seascapes in the world.

Mighty Tane Mahuta. Tane Mahuta, Lord of the Forest, whose palace is the splendid Waipoua Forest in Northland, is our largest kauri, towering above the lesser vegetation and selfie-snapping tourists with a regal tranquillity. It is estimated to be 2000, maybe even 2500, years old, meaning its seed first fell to earth around the time the pyramids were built at Giza, centuries before the Parthenon rose above Athens or Jesus of Nazareth preached in Palestine. I once read a fantasy story about a race of beings who, when they grew old and tired, found a favourite spot, put down roots and transformed into a tree. It sounded rather nice. When I visit Tane Mahuta I like to imagine it, too, possessing a sort of sentience filled with the wisdom of ages, which you can share if you open your mind.

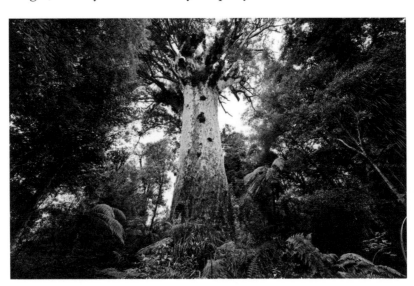

Waitangi Treaty Grounds. The Treaty Grounds evoke mixed emotions these days, I know . . . but have you actually been there? It's a stunning spot, with incredible views over the Bay of Islands, and there's the added charm of James Busby's house, the superbly carved meeting house and a magnificent war canoe. And then there's all that history. Sure, the treaty signed there was limited in its content and patchy in its application, but it was a pretty good effort by the standards of colonialism at the time and a better foundation than most countries can boast of. Visiting Waitangi gives me a sense of pride in the nation which sprang from this glorious birthplace.

Tiritiri Matangi. An island sanctuary in the Hauraki Gulf, Tiritiri Matangi allows visitors to get a feel for what the country was like before humans arrived to burn the forests and introduce rats and possums. As the sun rises, there's a dawn chorus of tuis and bellbirds, robins and kokako, to match the music of any orchestra. And, perhaps best of all, this is a place where over the past 50 years the grandchildren of settlers who cleared the island of bush and birds, making it an environmental desert, have reafforested it and reintroduced birds, to restore its glory. Tiritiri shows that what people have destroyed, people can repair.

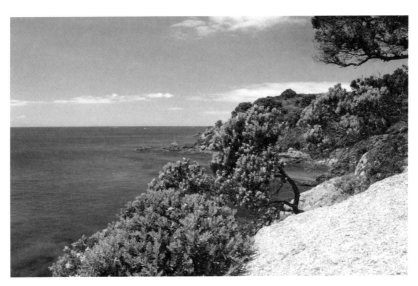

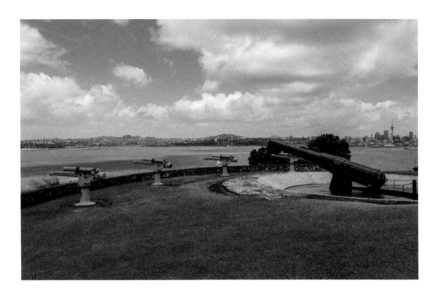

North Head, Devonport. North Head, Maungauika, the hill of Uika, offers spectacular views of central Auckland, from the golden sands of Cheltenham Beach and the islands of the Hauraki Gulf, to the busy port with its ships from around the world and the increasingly impressive skyline of the city centre. On days when there is yacht racing, with colourful spinnakers sending the boats flying through the water, it's a glorious sight. Maungauika also has a lot of history: Kupe the Discoverer, Toi the Navigator (most iwi believe that Uika, who built the first pa there, was Toi's brother) and the *Tainui* canoe are all said to have come ashore at its foot. Today it carries the earthworks, trenches, tunnels and guns left behind by centuries of fortifications designed to protect the area from Ngapuhi and Russian, Japanese and German invaders. It's endlessly fascinating to explore.

Miranda. On the shores of the Firth of Thames, Miranda is probably the best place in New Zealand to see the thousands of migratory shorebirds which gather here from afar. There's the little wrybill, up from the braided rivers of the South Island, the only bird in the world with a sideways bill. Or the bar-tailed godwits, red knots and

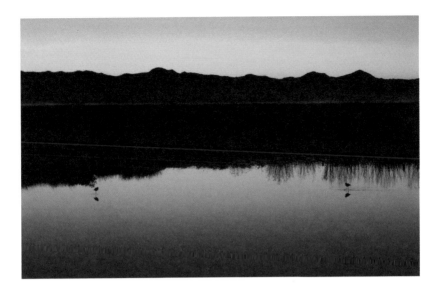

tiny red-necked stints, the size of a sparrow, which every year fly a 30,000km round trip from their homes in the Arctic. One godwit holds the world record for a non-stop long-distance flight, 11,760km direct from the Yukon Delta in Alaska to the mouth of the Piako River. Theirs is an extraordinary story. And watching the huge flocks as they soar and swirl, dip and dive above the shining mudflats and sparkling waves, the sun reflecting off their wings as if a giant silk scarf was waving in the sky, is an extraordinary experience.

Lake Tarawera. The lake is a gorgeous place in its own right, but its outlet is something extra special. Wander from the lake shore down the track along the beginnings of the Tarawera River and you'll notice lots of trout . . . and the fact that the river is slowly diminishing in size. Then, scarily, the last of the flow vanishes down a huge sinkhole, gurgling into the earth. Keep walking down the track, through a landscape which looks as though it never recovered from the eruption of nearby Mt Tarawera in 1886, and you'll see across the valley a massive cliff . . . with a river spouting out halfway down the rockface. The Tarawera River has emerged from the earth to resume its flow to the sea.

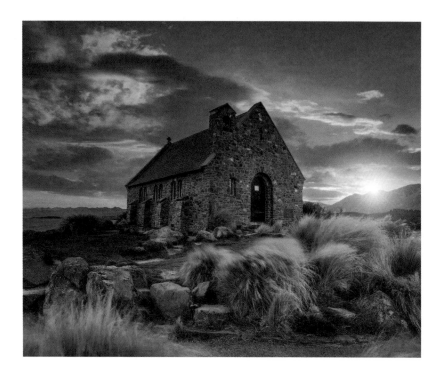

Church of the Good Shepherd, Lake Tekapo. You don't need to be religious to be moved by the sheer beauty of the Church of the Good Shepherd, on the shores of Lake Tekapo, high up in the Mackenzie Country. Built in 1935 from local stone, it fits perfectly into the landscape, and it must have the most glorious setting of any church. Beyond it, shining through the window behind the sanctuary, are the azure-blue waters of Lake Tekapo, and beyond the lake the soaring snow-capped peaks of the Southern Alps. At night the setting gets even better because the skies above are so clear they have been declared the Aoraki Mackenzie Dark Sky Reserve where, as one of the Psalms of David proclaims, 'The heavens declare the glory of God . . .'

Waitangiroto Nature Reserve, Whataroa, West Coast. The jetboat ride on the Waitangi Taona River is exciting enough, and the walk through the bush of the Waitangiroto Nature Reserve is a delight . . . but when you reach the hides at the end and gaze out at the trees on the opposite bank you start to marvel. This is the spot where each September–January every one of our 150–200 white heron, kotuku, put on their dancing clothes — long, wispy, white plumes — and come to court, mate, build nests and raise chicks. They're surely our most elegant birds and watching them perform in this unique and lovely spot is an absolute joy.

Dusky Sound. Visit Dusky Sound on a classic misty Fiordland day, with clouds rolling down the thickly forested slopes and the cliffs glittering with waterfalls, and you could easily imagine that you've gone back in time to some primeval era before humans existed. But, while it may seem untouched, in fact it contains some of the earliest signs of Europeans in New Zealand. On the southeast shore is the spot where in 1773 Captain James Cook set up camp for three months, repairing his ship, replenishing food supplies and — perhaps most significant of all — brewing the first beer made in this country. You can even see the stump of a huge tree felled to create a platform for an astronomical observatory. Sit in the silence of the mist and it's all too easy to imagine his ghostly crew going about the work which, in the end, would transform these islands.

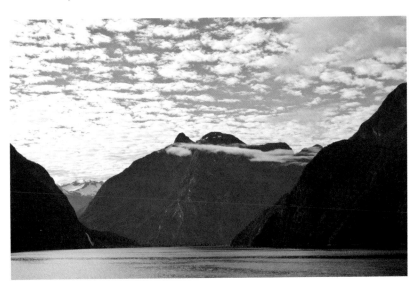

Sexual Issues
Everlasting Love

Locker-room talk got a whole new meaning when Donald Trump claimed sexual assault was a common topic when the boys got together. Australian writer Peter FitzSimons, having been in many changing sheds as a test rugby player, spoke for a lot of us when he said that, in fact, when normal guys actually talked amongst themselves 'mostly the preening turns on how attractive your most recent partner is, with the goal being to demonstrate what a slick bloke I must be to pull such a chick as this, "Don't you reckon, guys?!" And the second strand is even more gauche, boasting how many attractive women you've pulled, hence how super slick you must be. "Don'tcha reckon youse blokes, you guys?"'

It's not that men won't mention their penis to other men. We even have our own names for it, like the old fella, the wife's best friend, John Thomas, Mr Wobbly, the one-eyed trouser snake, Willy, the Y-fronts piccolo, donger, or Percy, as in 'point Percy at the porcelain'.

But what's even more super, dead set, 100% guaranteed is that bloke conversations will never turn to failure to rise in bed, aka erectile dysfunction, or being trigger happy while having sex, aka premature ejaculation. If we ever did talk honestly about them, we'd be amazed at how common they were. Forget the way dicks like Trump talk, if you're having some issues with love making you're far from alone.

At 40, estimates the highly respected Cleveland Clinic in Ohio, about 40 per cent of men have a problem getting an erection and at 70 the number increases to 70%.

Premature ejaculation? University of Chicago studies of 2865 men in 1999 and 2008 found that around 30% of men from the age of 18 to 74 were concerned about how quickly they came.

Jan Burns is an expert in the field. A registered nurse since 1993, she has a degree in sexual therapy from the University of Sydney, and has worked and studied further in the United States. She says it's an unfortunate fact that in New Zealand there's very little education about men's sexual issues. 'Advertising is still very limited, and so awareness is limited, too, and that's very sad because you do need that normalisation to occur, so men get the confidence to know it's not such a difficult conversation.'

There are very successful, proven medical ways to deal with performance issues, but for a lot of us it's still not easy to pluck up the courage and make the walk from our home to a doctor's surgery. The great news is that the payoff may astound you. You will be treated with decency and courtesy. And there is help out there that actually works.

Now based at the Virtuoso Clinic in Tauranga, Jan Burns says, 'A lot of men bluff their way through when they're actually hurting. There is a perception in our society that men have to be tough and strong. Don't cry and be the bread-winner. But men hurt just like everybody else. I've seen marriages break down, partners walk away because it's just got too difficult. I have seen various degrees of depression and suicidal tendencies.'

The sad thing is it doesn't have to be that way. Yes, as Jan says, for many Kiwi men to speak about sexual dysfunction is a courageous conversation. But with 22 years of experience to go by, she says 99% of GPs men approach will be 'absolutely positive and can implement a treatment plan'.

She has one piece of advice for a guy taking the first step to getting back on the 'sexual track', and that's to make at least the initial visit to your doctor a solo one. 'It's more difficult with a partner, because a man will fear he may upset the partner in some way. Or the partner may feel he no longer finds her attractive because they're having erectile dysfunction, or intimacy issues. In my own assessments I prefer to talk to the man first, and then the couple, if they are a couple.'

As well as being sympathetic, the other advantage of seeing a GP is that the advice you get will be accurate. 'Some men turn to Dr Google on the net for electronic education,' says Jan, 'and some of that can be very misleading. It sets them up for failure because they have unrealistic expectations.'

It may help to look at what actually happens when the penis stands up for sex, and why sometimes it doesn't.

Basically, says urologist Chris Hawke, the penis works as a hydraulic ram. 'There are two main chambers inside the shaft that at the base splay out in a Y shape (called the crura), and attach to the underside of the pubic arch. If you look at the pelvis from the front, there's a ridge of bone they attach to. Those two chambers pump up under the right kind of provocation and inside a tough outer casing is very spongy tissue. It has got lots of spaces within it that blood can fill. A message goes from the brain, via the spine, via pelvic nerves, into the spongy penile tissue, the arteries open up, blood pours into those spaces, and pumps up the tyre, so to speak.'

So far, so straightforward. As most of us can remember, sometimes with acute embarrassment if asked to stand up in class, that 'right kind of provocation' when you're a teenager can be as basic as the replacement English teacher being a buxom woman in her 20s.

When everything is functioning, something very clever happens to the veins in the penis, which are almost all on the outside. They're on an angle and, as blood pouring into the spongy chambers inside inflates the penis, the veins get squeezed, and they shut, not allowing any blood out. Voila! First step to erection.

Second step? What's called a skeleton erection. Or, in teenage medical terms, a woody. 'There are also some muscles that wrap around the base of the penis,' says Chris, 'that are partly there for ejaculatory reasons, and are also partly there because they can tighten up even more, and make the pressure inside the penis go really quite high. It is called the stage of skeletal erection, where the penis is very hard. Now, it is that woody hardness that guys will tend to lose with aging. The vascular mechanism is still working, but the muscles around the base of the penis aren't giving them the same sort of extreme hardness.'

What causes things to go wrong? It's a broad spread. It may be a side effect of prostate treatment, either with surgery or radiation. Some medications can cause difficulties with erections. Recreational drugs might be a problem.

'There may be some age-related slight arterial disease going on,' says Chris Hawke. 'The penile tissue itself is getting older, and there is a combination of mild deficits that together cause a problem.

'Smoking is a big, identifiable factor. Smoking causes arterial constriction. It is the most potent cause of vascular disease known to man, so to speak, and it is probably the easiest remedial cause for erectile dysfunction. So if you are a middle-aged guy who still smokes, and your erection is not working so well, stop smoking.'

It can also be, says Jan Burns, a loss of self-esteem and confidence, so that intimacy becomes something a man avoids.

When all's well with the penis, and sexual arousal starts, there's a chemical chain that causes the arteries to open up, blood to flow in, and an erection to pop up. To switch it off later there's also an enzyme that closes things up, so the erection doesn't last all day. Call it the off switch.

The biggest change in treatment, the material for a million comedians, and a godsend for a lot more men, arrived with Viagra and similar drugs, such as Levitra and Cialis. They came about almost by accident.

'A drug company had a compound on trial, because it was mildly effective for treating high blood pressure and some other cardiovascular conditions,' says Chris. 'At the end of the trial period the patients weren't keen to give their tablets back, because it was giving their erectile function a boost. These were guys that were on a blood pressure-type trial; they were older guys with high blood pressure who often had high cholesterol and a bit of diabetes as well.

'The good thing about Viagra, and its sister drugs, is the way they work, which is by blocking the "off" enzyme in the penis. This enzyme is present in very few other parts of the body in significant amounts. So it has very little effect on the rest of the body. You get some mild flushing of the face, and it can make white light look slightly blueish, because it affects an enzyme in the retina. But, overall, the side effects are mild.

'Once you get to a certain age it basically winds the clock back about ten years. It just gives your natural mechanism a boost.'

Online, and on air, there are numerous other treatments advertised for erectile dysfunction. Jan Burns is one who doesn't mince words about the miracle cures. 'When I screen my patients I'm very black and white. If I think they're going to spend $300 on something that I know won't work I will tell them that. They don't have to listen to me, but I tell them that in my two decades of experience I have never seen this product work. I've done my own research and I don't believe it will work for you. I do lay it on the line and 99% of the time they are very grateful.'

In plain terms, Jan Burns and Chris Hawke suggest that whatever treatment you're thinking of, whether it's mail-order pills or self-proclaimed specialists in the field, check it out with your GP first. If in doubt ask a medical professional you trust.

Viagra, and its sister drugs, do work, but what they can't promise is erections for life. There are more radical options available if the Viagra rise starts to flag.

'If Viagra is not working, for whatever reason, you can use an injectable drug that skips the nerves altogether,' says Chris Hawke. 'You are injecting something into the penal tissue that will cause the smooth muscle to relax and the blood vessels to open up and you will get an erection.'

Just back up the truck a second! You inject your own penis? Yes.

The needles are as small as those used by people with diabetes, that is, about one-third the length of an eyelash and of extremely narrow diameter. There's no other way to say this: it'll only be a little prick.

Jan Burns has comforting words. 'Men cringe at the thought of injections but, in fact, when you know how to do it, it's not painful and it gives the most stunning erections, that many thought they might never see again. Some of my patients are in tears at how good the results are.

'The trade-off is that you lose the spontaneity because sex becomes very much a planned thing. But when you think about it, it was always planned in your head. "What kind of day has my wife had? Are the kids around?" You were always planning it, but now you have to verbally plan it. You have to ask, "Shall we try the injection tonight?" Sometimes I think guys need to hear from a medical person that it's perfectly okay to think and talk like that.'

Rather than fear of needles, says Chris Hawke, a more important element with injections is making sure you get the dose right. The best way to ensure this, he says, is to start with your GP, making sure you're being referred to an experienced and reputable specialist.

The wrong dose can lead to a condition called priapism, where an erection won't go down. It sounds like a 20-year-old guy's greatest fantasy, but in fact, because blood won't flow back out of the penis, something that usually happens naturally with orgasm, the lack of blood flow inside the penis can damage the spongy tissues as cells die, and eventually cause permanent problems with erections.

Another aid is a vacuum pump that fits over the penis, and helps to draw blood into it, which is then held in by a ring around the penis' base. 'It's probably not great as a standalone option,' says Chris, 'but if someone has had a major prostate operation I can get him to use it as well as Viagra to maximise the chances of a full recovery.'

If Viagra, vacuum pumps, and injections don't do the job there is one more procedure, increasingly popular in America, still quite rare here. It's called an implantable penial prosthesis. Think of it as an artificial hip for your penis. Under a full anaesthetic cylinders are inserted into the two chambers filled with spongy tissue inside the penis. The artificial cylinders are connected by tubing to a pump inside your scrotum. The pump connects to a fluid reservoir that is usually buried inside your abdomen. When everything heals, it all looks exactly as it did before the operation.

The pump is activated by pushing on the button inside your scrotum. It's much the same process as pushing a button on a Buzz Lightyear toy to make him talk. Your penis doesn't say 'To Infinity and beyond' but it does rise up.

'You've got a penis that erects when you pump it up,' says Chris. 'It feels warm, and lifelike. It is not like some inanimate dildo. It is a living penis that is inflated artificially. So it can give you a virtually normal quality erection when you want it.

'If you're a guy in his 70s who wants to have sex once a month, you know, it is not worth it. Maybe injections or a combination of Viagra and a vacuum pump, or maybe you are just over it. But for someone who has had, say, bladder cancer, and is 45 and neither he nor his wife want to be celibate for the rest of their lives, for the right guy this is a very good option.'

Billy T James (in a giggly voice): 'Hey, do you know why most Australian men are premature ejaculators?'
Billy T (straight voice): 'No. Why are most Australian men premature ejaculators?'
Billy T (giggly): 'Because they just can't wait to tell the boys!'

In the song 'December 1963 (Oh What a Night)' Frankie Valli and the Four Seasons sang, 'And I felt a rush like a rolling bolt of thunder/ Spinning my head around and taking my body under/Oh, what a night/ . . . As I recall, it ended much too soon.'

How soon is too soon once a penis is inside a vagina? An international group of sexual experts in 2014 suggested anything under three minutes was an issue, others suggest two minutes or 60 seconds.

More to the point, says Chris Hawke, it isn't what the stopwatch says, but a persistent inability to delay coming that you find annoying, or worse, or isn't satisfactory for your partner. 'Your ability to hold back ejaculation is kind of intrinsic. Some guys are very ticklish and some are not, some people are very jumpy and some aren't. It is just the way you are.'

But if you, or your partner, is unhappy with what's happening it doesn't have to continue to be that way. Historically there's been the folklore that suggested you think of cricket to slow things down while having sex. That might have worked in the stately days of test cricket, but could be a problem in the Big Bash, wham bam, quick-fire style of the game now. Sex researchers Masters and Johnson introduced a technique in the 1970s which involved having your partner squeeze your penis just under the glans, or head, as you were close to ejaculating.

'There was also waiting, and then going again,' says Chris. 'Neither was terribly satisfactory. The reflexes that control ejaculation have become better understood, and from a therapeutic point of view there are some local things you can do.

'You can slather the penis in local anaesthetic-type creams, or use condoms that have got a local anaesthetic built into the lube. Those things can work to a degree. Or else you can take medication.'

Drugs can help with premature ejaculation. There are basically two types that can be prescribed. One is to be prescribed a low dose of an antidepressant, such as Prozac or Fluoxetine. 'They tend to have fewer sedating side effects than older antidepressant drugs, but one thing that is a common side effect of these drugs is either retardation or complete elimination of ejaculation. They can also impair your libido (or sex drive). But assuming the libido is strong, if premature ejaculation is a problem, then taking a low dose of one of these drugs can be useful.'

There's also an antidepressant drug called Priligy. 'It has a short half-life, so you take it, and half an hour to an hour later you are good to go for lasting longer than otherwise would be the case. The next morning it is out of your system. Whether you're using that, or a daily low dose of antidepressants, it's something to talk to your GP about.'

* * *

If you Google 'sexual function and/or performance' you'll get everything from porn sites to shonky pills and potions to buy. The extensive Ministry of Health website, health.govt.nz/your-health, doesn't mention sexual performance issues. In this case it's best to leave the net and visit your doctor.

The fact the Ministry of Health's website doesn't mention sexual function is reflected in the fact that while, as an example, women who have undergone a mastectomy are, quite rightly, offered financial help with prosthetic breasts, men who have had a major prostate operation are offered no public funding for treatment that can restore sexual function. 'Treatment for men often comes down to a matter of cost,' says Jan Burns, 'and I think that's very sad.'

Exercise
Finding Your Fun

Nic Gill has been the All Blacks' strength and conditioning coach since 2008. Enthusiastic and energetic, he's the sort of guy Barry Crump would have called a good keen man. He's passionate about the All Blacks, but meet Nic and you soon find he's just as passionate about helping Kiwi blokes to get fit and healthy.

Kids exercise because it's fun. They call it playing. One of the first things we can do as adults about our fitness is to find out what exercise we enjoy. We should cast that net wide. Find something you enjoy, and it'll never be a chore. If you exercise just because you think you should, there's a very good chance you won't enjoy it, and you won't do it for long.

I spend a lot of my working life with the All Blacks in gyms. But, here's a confession, I don't especially like lifting weights any more. On the other hand, I love digging holes, pushing a wheelbarrow, digging a trench, or mowing the lawns. You can guess what I tend to do the most of in my own time.

Your exercise bliss may be something quite different. If it's gym work, great. You might like doing stuff with a group of mates. Do you like going for jogs along the beach, walking through the bush, or do you like playing touch rugby?

The most important thing is that if you find something you have some fun with, you'll always be wanting to do it.

Our aim? It may not be winning a Rugby World Cup, or making

a 1500 metres final at the Olympics, but we can all have our own, hugely important goal: being fit for life. Fit for life means being fit and healthy for as long as possible, so you can get the most out of your day, your family and your work.

It's worth taking a little time to think about what sparks your interest, and it could start by having a good look right at home.

Finding out if you're a Floater or an Energiser Bunny

Let's look first at what sort of person you are when it comes to exercise. Knowing what drives you will be a big help in making decisions. Most of us break down into four types:

The Watcher. He hates exercise, so is largely inactive, and likely to be in worse shape than anyone else.

The Floater. A lot of us are floaters. For a week or two we get into exercise, but then lose interest and start doing nothing.

The Energiser Bunny. He just loves being active. His reward comes from the good feelings the dopamine his exercise produces flood his body with.

The Challenger. He gets his buzz from taking on something and achieving his goal. A perfect example in this country? Sir Edmund Hillary.

Understanding where you fit should help you figure out what it is you need to find.

It's not a matter of doing exercise just for the sake of doing exercise, if you want it to become part of your life then you need to legitimately enjoy some aspects of it. Whether it's enjoying how it makes you feel, whether it's enjoying how it makes you look, or whether it is a matter of enjoying what it allows you to eat, it doesn't really matter.

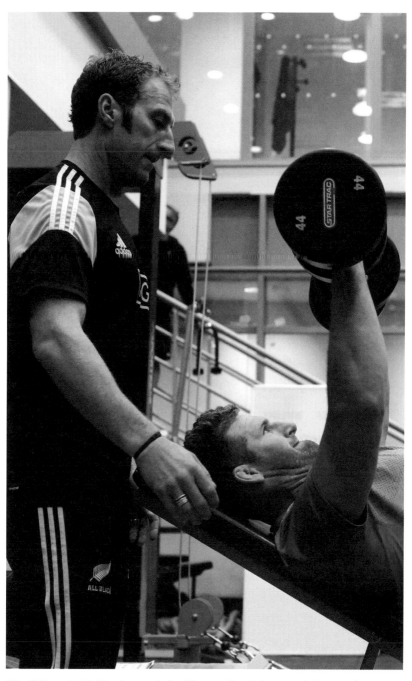

Nic Gill and All Blacks captain Kieran Read in a training environment that works for the All Blacks. Others may work better for you.

For me, I love a challenge and I love food. So I need a challenge and part of the challenge is allowing me to eat the lovely food that is a huge part of my day. So I think identifying the type of person you are, or the type of structure you need to be able to be active, is very important.

What should suit me if I'm a Watcher?

First of all, it's okay to not love exercise, it's okay to not have a training programme, and it's okay to not go to the gym.

But there are many other ways to be active during the day. One is to look at what you might call incidentals. Maybe parking your car three blocks from work and walking. Walking up the stairs to the fifth floor instead of taking the lift. Finding the stairs at the mall or airport and using them instead of the escalator.

Building up your levels of activity is not an impossible dream. What needs to be kept in mind are the benefits you get from regular exercise.

Every minute of every day cells are dying, and living cells are being replicated. As soon as you stop, within a couple of days, the body is starting to pull back on what it needs to be able to do. Those cells are being replicated based on what they've experienced, or the body has experienced, over the last 24/36/48 hours. Just sitting, the muscle in our body is turning over. But if you don't use it, you lose it. Use it and you'll get to that state that all of us would like to live our life in, jumping out of bed in the morning, looking forward to a great day, and looking back on the great week we've just had.

If you keep stressing the cells a little, or adding exercise, you will keep being healthier and fitter day by day, week by week.

At one stage I used to think that if I went for one really good run a week I would be fine. Doesn't happen. Exercise needs to be regular, and often, and consistent.

A realistic health guide is 20 to 30 minutes of exercise, three or four times a week.

It is consistent. It is not overdoing it. Just a little bit here and there to remind the body you need to be able to jump on that bike for half an hour, you need to be able to climb those stairs, you need to be able to walk around that park, you need to be able to mow the lawns.

Later we'll talk about some ideas around eating that I'm sure can help you if you're a watcher.

What will work if I'm a Floater?

You're a relaxed sort of person and exercise isn't a chore, but it's not a really big buzz or a driver, it is just something that is okay to fit in when you can. You don't mind exercise, you quite enjoy mowing the lawns, or going for a brisk walk. But you'll only do it when you feel like it, and that may not be that often.

What can you do to make it regular, fun and hugely helpful? A great way is to make your exercise part of your social life. For most of us, if we are just doing it by ourselves, it is easy to put exercise off. 'I'm not going to have time today.' It's easy to come up with an excuse or a reason for it to not happen.

But let's say you join a touch footy team, or a social netball side. You can't let other people down. If you know your mates will be there you'll get there too. And if there are other people involved, they not only get you to the point of doing it, but it's also much more fun. If you make a social connection with your exercise, that's awesome.

A great way to float exercise in and out of your life (but consistently) is with work colleagues or family. Instead of sitting in an office talking media strategy, advertising budgets, or staff issues, go for a walk through the city, or around the park, and 'talk and walk'. The same goes for your loved ones. Instead of texting each other, living through technology, take your daughter or son for a walk/jog through the bush or park.

What's best for the Energiser man?

You're fortunate if the reward from exercise is the exercise itself. Typically, for the active person, exercise is a little bit like a drug: it is the feeling, the daily buzz of endorphins.

The benefits of exercise for our mental and physical wellbeing are enormous. If you're our energiser man you already know that, so the only area you need to consider is that whatever physical activity you're doing, you're not feeling broken at the end of it.

Ideally you would go for a walk and you would have a stretch and you would feel great. Or you would go for a bike ride and you would get off the bike and you are just, 'Man, that was so cool, I enjoyed that. I feel great.'

Gyms are exactly the same: you should be able to walk into a gym, do some exercise, and walk out feeling a million dollars.

When you walk out feeling like you have been beaten up, it becomes a major barrier to continued health and being fit for life. You need to keep your body healthy, free from injury, and free from aches and pains.

But if you constantly feel really good from doing what you are doing, then that is positive reinforcement, and nothing will stand in your way!

How do challenges help?

Some guys really rise to a challenge, so it can be a terrific way to make you want to exercise.

I have a group of mates, and we identify a trip each year, and we say, 'Okay, let's go and run over the Tongariro Crossing.' What we enjoy is that we're doing it together as a group of mates and we're using that to get ourselves fitter and healthier.

We are almost like a team scattered around the country, and we're worried about letting the other guys down, so we make sure we get out there and do our runs in the middle of winter.

Some people react well to identifying something that scares them. I do Ironman, and that scares me. But it gets me out of bed when I don't want to get out of bed, and I go and exercise.

I rode 250km on my bike the other day. Someone said, 'Why?' I said, 'Because I haven't ridden 250km on my bike before.'

That's my thing, a challenge. But people have to find their thing. The thing that is going to add to their mental and physical health. Because having something to think about that is not just work and money is important. So you come back from a session feeling, 'Wow, I'm stoked I did that. I feel great, I feel confident, I feel like I could take on the world.'

With challenges come rewards, and they don't have to be as dramatic as the satisfaction of finishing something as demanding as an Ironman.

Having a more active life gives you more freedom to enjoy better food. And being able to have a couple of beers whenever you want because you are doing a bit of exercise is pretty rewarding too.

Planning your day to feel good

We book in going to work, or picking up kids from school, or going to a movie or out for a meal, or getting a warrant for our car.

If you do exactly the same with exercise I promise it'll become much easier. It needs to have a specific place in your day, whether that's in your lunch break, before work, after work, or in the weekend, you need to book it in, otherwise it's the last thing to happen.

Prioritise it and six months won't have somehow gone by without you doing any activity, feeling horrible and having no energy.

If you prioritise some activity then you won't have the feelings of low energy, you won't have the fluctuations in mood, you won't feel like you need to eat more because you just crave sugar. Book exercise in, and it'll happen.

Something I find worth considering also is the fact that if I wait until the end of the day to exercise it is less likely to happen. But if I start my day with exercise I never have to go through the mind games of 'Should I?' 'Nah, I can't be bothered.' 'Go on, you'll feel better.' 'Nah, I'll just go tomorrow.'

Making your own timetable

I believe everything is trainable. A lot of people say they can't exercise in the morning. To me it's just a matter of quietly taking maybe three months to build up to it, and then it'll feel normal. I don't mind exercising at three or four in the afternoon but, let's be honest, then I've got a whole day of excuses to come up with before I get to three or four.

That's where most people come undone. They feel, 'Today has just been such a big day at work, I'm not going to exercise tonight.' It is a big barrier for a lot of people. It is the day getting in the way.

But everything with our body is trainable. And not just our body clocks. I eat peanut butter when I'm running now. I take a little squeezy thing of peanut butter with me. Ten years ago there is no way I could have done that. But my body has been trained to digest it, and it's great.

The rewards of keeping on

Sometimes people think that as we get older we need to do more exercise. We shouldn't need to do more, but we should continue what we've been doing. Often, when we get older we slow down, and we stop doing things that we used to do, because we think we should because we're older.

But we don't need to stop. The healthy older men out there are the ones that are still working the land, or still riding bikes, or still walking, or still being active. As soon as we stop or as soon as we slow down, the body adapts or reacts to that. I think it's important to remember that if you use it, you don't lose it.

What's the best exercise when you hit your 40s?

The decade from age 40 to 50 is an interesting one because typically most men at that age have a little bit more time on their hands, because your kids have grown up, or the career is booming because it has taken 20 years to establish yourself in your niche, and where you are going.

Maybe you have got more disposable income. Everyone is different.

But the 40s is definitely that point where most men sit back and go, 'Holy crap, I need to get fit, I need to get healthy, I need to sort my health out.'

If I was asked to say what is most important, the best exercise, my answer would be, 'I don't think it matters as long as you're doing something.'

Whether you're walking, jogging, sprinting, surfing, cycling, hiking, hunting, lifting weights, going to yoga classes, stretching, or doing little circuits in your bedroom, as long as you're doing something there will be huge benefits downstream.

We also need to adjust to workloads and seasonal changes. Be realistic. Winter is tough.

The body, as we get older, can cope with everything we could do when we were younger, but we tend to be a little more delicate when it comes to big changes like running hard, or longer, or lifting something a little heavier than we have for a while. This is the key change that occurs with age.

Maybe we are not as durable as we were, BUT we are just as capable, if we're smart, our exercise is progressive, and things are not dramatically changed in short periods of time. People try to look for the silver bullet, the one thing that is going to make a difference, and it doesn't exist. It is a matter of consistently doing something, being active and keeping the body moving.

Starting all over again

You're fired up, you've made a resolution to get fit again and, quite often, within two weeks you've hurt yourself. Whatever you do, ease into it slowly. Think about being consistent, and make your exercise plan one that initially involves exercise that's small and often.

Personally, I go through about two months of niggles and injuries getting fit, if I have a period of intensive work, and minimal consistent exercise. No matter what I've done in the past, it takes me a couple of months to build up to where I want to be.

We all have injuries from the past, aches and pains and restrictions. So easing into things and creating habits and a routine is more important than trying to figure out what is the one big thing that you need to do.

Let's get specific about the gym

I'm 41 now, and if I was going to the gym for the first time, or after a lengthy break, I would be wanting to make sure that I do a little bit of mobility and stretching to loosen up the creaky joints, to warm the muscles up, to regain some of that useful movement.

Then I would be looking to do some resistance training and movements that don't hurt any of my joints, so using machines and free weights to resist movement is really important.

Then I would finish with some cardiovascular-type exercise, something to get the heart rate up, more so than the weights. So you are strengthening muscle, and you strengthen bone and the cardiovascular system.

To end the session, I would have a stretch and a recovery session, maybe a massage.

So, we've done our weights, we've done our aerobic or cardiovascular work, we've done our stretching and mobility, and then we've done what we needed to do at the end to walk out feeling a million bucks!

Why does stretching matter?

Typically, from when we are born we have a great range of motion in our hips, knees, ankles, shoulders and spine. As we become more inactive as we get older, we stop using movement and we start losing movement in our hips, we start getting sore backs, we start getting creaky knees, and our ankles ache if we run. It is mainly because we have stopped going through those ranges of motion, so we have lost that range.

Stretching shouldn't just be about stretching a muscle, it should be taking joints through ranges of motion that we used to be able to do.

So squatting with a straight back so the hips are taken through a full range is just as important as stretching or lengthening the hamstrings. We need to make sure that the mobility, or the functional movement, is given as much attention as the longer muscles.

Machines or free weights?

I'd suggest you start with machines. Build up a little bit of a training history with machine weights and then, when you're feeling confident and competent, get some guidance or ask to train with someone to take you through the correct use of free weights.

Free weights will be better in the long term, but there's a little more risk of injury at the start, because you can go through ranges or positions that aren't anatomically correct and then you hurt yourself.

With time, though, you'll get better progress using free weights, because you're not restricted in the range of movements, as you are by a machine.

What other machines are good?

The cross trainers are great; the rowers, elliptical trainers, bikes, treadmills, steppers, all those things are great.

The joy of the gym when you're older comes from the things that you can do without pounding and smashing your joints. You get the cardiovascular benefits without your hips, knees and ankles suffering.

Rowing machines are fantastic. But, it is like anything, rowers are great as long as you've got good form. As long as you have got a nice strong back and you are not overloading something that shouldn't be loaded. The bikes are the same, the treadmills are the same. As long as you've got reasonably good function and technique, they are amazing.

The good thing about elliptical trainers is that while they work both the arms and the legs, there is no impact, so people who can't run can use them without causing any damage.

How to start jogging

Running is tough. Jogging is an area that's probably the best bang for your buck, but it's also probably the highest-risk exercise for older people. Easing into things is most important for this particular exercise.

When you run, you've got your full bodyweight landing on one foot with a bit of momentum. So the stress on the muscles and joints is quite large. Especially as we get heavier. If we're carrying a few extra kilos, then the stress is magnified four-six-tenfold.

My advice, if you want to start jogging after not doing a lot, is to always run or jog at a speed where you can talk. If you're running at a speed where you can talk, then your fitness will dictate how fast you go and it will limit how long you can run for.

So, for example, most 50-year-old men, if they hadn't been running for several years, they'd have to run very slowly to still hold a conversation, and they might only be able to jog for five minutes when they begin. Your body will tell you what works without hurting yourself.

A magic way to get back into jogging

A phenomenal thing to do for anyone wanting to just be healthy without any particular goal in mind, just wanting to be active, is walk jogging.

You break it up with some walking. You might start off with a two-minute jog and a two-minute walk. It might be one to one. It might be a one-minute jog, a three-minute walk. You're just jogging a little bit at a time. Then, every week or two, very slowly, you increase the amount of jogging that you do.

Why is this so great? Number one: you actually enjoy it, because it is not too hard. Number two: the likelihood of injuring yourself is reduced significantly. Number three: because of those two points, you are likely to make it a habit you'll make time for. And number four could be: you can have conversations and catch up with people.

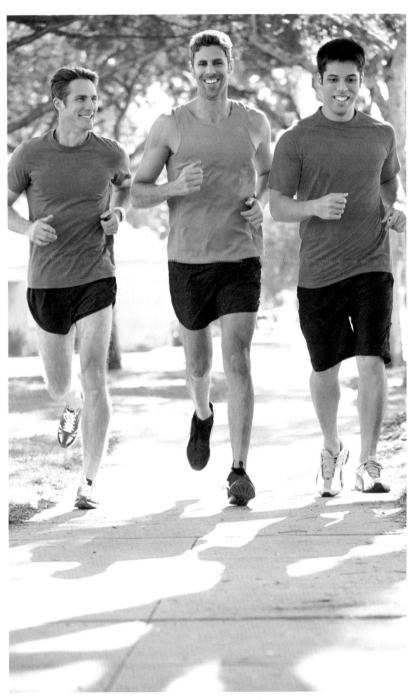

If you exercise with other people involved it's much more fun.

I do it with my daughter. She picks a time that we are going to jog and a time we are going to walk. So the other night we did five-two, a five-minute jog and a two-minute walk. We did that for 40 minutes. What it means is that you can break up the exercise, as a lot of people can't continuously jog for 20 or 30 or 40 minutes.

We have 40 minutes together every second day that otherwise I don't have. I don't need the jog, but it is great for her and it is teaching her lifelong habits about being healthy. The thing I love about it is we talk non-stop for 40 minutes. There is nothing else, except me and her, and it is great. So more people should be looking at doing this. Doing this with husbands and wives, sons and daughters, mates. Anyone can do it.

Be kind to your joints when you run

Once you start running a lot you'll find a huge difference between running on concrete footpaths and roads, and running on softer surfaces like grass or bush tracks. Do all your running on the road and the next day you'll be stiff and sore. If you've had a long run on grass your muscles will be tired, but that's all.

The other thing with running on roads is that they're cambered. So often people start getting a sore knee or a sore ankle because they are running on an angle the whole time. Usually it is always the same way, because you go down one side of the road, facing traffic, and you come back on the other side of the road. The right foot that was low going out is still low coming back.

Getting off concrete has another benefit too. If you're on a softer surface, the views and the environment are usually that much better. You're in the bush or in a park and it is so much nicer. So it is not only so much better for the joints, but it is also better for the soul.

Off-season training isn't just for All Blacks

Social team sport is awesome. It's fun, you're out there doing it, and you're enjoying being competitive. But to make sure you make the most of it, you do need to prepare for it. If you don't, the results won't be flash. I know five people in their early 40s who have ruptured their Achilles tendons playing social netball.

When we're 18 we can do almost anything without real preparation. But as you get older, then about a month before the season starts you need to do some training to cut down the chance of a major injury.

Don't let the whole point of what you're doing be lost because of injury. Invest some time in getting your body ready for what you're going to put it through, and then have the time of your life when you play.

FOOD
Eating what you burn

Most of us would be lying if we said we didn't like food. If you're from the generation, like me, whose fathers and grandfathers worked the land, building fences and doing hard physical jobs, you'll probably have been brought up with the idea that a big piece of steak, a big pile of potatoes, and a few peas will get you through.

But we're not as active as a lot of those men in previous generations.

It's important that we learn that and get the balance right between what we're eating and what we're burning. The biggest weight problem in New Zealand, and in many countries, is created when people's nutritional intake stays the same, but activity levels drop. So they put on weight. And with kids spending more time at computers and less time outside, we're seeing it happen earlier.

It can be difficult to get your head around it at first, but once you understand it, it's pretty simple.

The good news: it tastes better if you've earned it

If you're exercising you can have more flexibility with your food and drink. It might be that you love a cold beer at the end of a hot day, or a lovely pinot noir with dinner. Nothing wrong with that. But remember, you need to have 'earned' it first.

I think exercising helps your discipline around how you eat. If

I don't train on a particular day, my self-control and discipline to eat well goes. I reckon it's that reward thing. If I exercise, my body is happy. Then if I'm not exercising, my body is saying, 'You need something to make you feel good.' I want comfort.

I love good-quality dark chocolate. When I'm exercising I'll have a row of chocolate. There's no harm done. But what doesn't make any logical sense is that when I'm not exercising, and should actually be cutting back, I'll eat four rows, or even a whole bar. That's my body talking, not my mind. I've learned that about myself, and we all need to understand ourselves, and how our body reacts to exercise, or the lack of it.

If you have a couple of beers, or sometimes enjoy a pie, that's fine. Just as long as you've been digging a gutter, or walked the beach, or run around the block, or tramped in the bush. That pie? Enjoy it, but keep in mind you really need to have jogged for 30 or 40 minutes to burn it off. If you haven't been for a jog? Maybe you shouldn't have it.

That's the simple question you should be asking yourself: In the last 24 hours, have I just been sitting at a computer or in a car? If I have, then I need to cut back on how much I eat.

I am not an advocate of telling people not to have a beer, because I think if you enjoy drinking a beer why can't you have it if you have earned it? What's really important is understanding that having one Steinlager Pure takes you 25 minutes of walking a dog to get rid of.

If you're just thirsty and you haven't been for that 25-minute walk, have water. But if you have been for your walk and you are thirsty, you'd love a beer, you've had a good day, and you just want to sit back and chill out with your partner, then you understand that it is fine to have it.

It's not a diet; it's eating colourfully

Dieting is always a short-term fix and so many studies show that, over time, diets never work. What we're talking about here is eating well for life, which goes hand in hand with exercise. In other words, a lifestyle that gives you a fuller, happier life.

Let's look at ways that will help you get the vitamins and minerals you need. A great way to start is to have lots of bright colours on your plate. If you look at colourful foods such as tomato, carrot, cabbage, or avocado, they're full of nutrients, vitamins and minerals. They're very, very good for you.

And here's the big bonus: they're generally reasonably low in calories too. So if you want to fill up, eat the colourful foods that have got all the good stuff in them, and go easy on the other stuff.

On the other hand, it's worth trying to reduce the amount of dull, white-coloured food you eat. I'm talking about rice, bread, pasta and potatoes. The ones with lots of carbohydrates.

Why is it so worthwhile to try to cut back on the dull foods? If you have, let's say, four pieces of toast for breakfast, you are starting your day by adding a lot of calories, but very few nutrients.

Consuming more calories than your body needs, whether from carbohydrates, protein, or fats, means they will be stored as fat. So if you eat too much protein, from overdoing meat in your diet, or even, theoretically, colourful vegetables, you can get fat.

But it's much harder to overeat with the good stuff, especially with good vegetables.

Let me give you an example. One cup of cooked white rice has about the same number of calories as four to five cups of broccoli. If I have four cups of broccoli in my curry I'm going to leave the table a lot more satisfied than if I've had one measly cup of rice, and I've had my daily intake of vitamins A and C.

Balancing the plate

Back in the day, and I'm thinking about the 60s, 70s and 80s, a Kiwi bloke's dinner at night at home was often three or four sausages, a pile of mashed spuds, and a few peas.

We used to be a country where a lot of people had physical jobs. As an example, in 1963–64 on an All Blacks tour of Britain, six of the eight men in the test forward pack were, or had been, farmers.

If you're working hard, throwing in some carbs is fine. But if you're not burning them up, they'll be stored in the body as fat.

Today, in general, as Kiwi blokes, we tend to have too many carbs for the amount of exercise we do, so we get fatter over time.

And with kids spending time with computers, rather than running around outside, we see the problems with weight happening earlier.

If you balance what's on your plate, so that at least half of it is colourful foods, and a quarter of it protein, you're cutting down the white starchy carbs, from the likes of potatoes.

Look above the ground

Any vegetable that's exposed to the sun the whole time is full of nutrients and colour. The stuff that grows underneath is typically a bit duller, a bit whiter.

We want to reduce how much of that we have. It is still real food, and it has still got benefits, but we should be careful not to overdo it.

Let's compare, for example, broccoli and potatoes. Broccoli is high in vitamins and it is not energy, or calorie, dense. But a potato, while high in vitamins and minerals, has around twice the calories.

Both broccoli and potatoes are real food, but in general terms, the vegetables that live in the sun and fresh air are better for us. You're trying to have a plate that provides longer-lasting, quality energy.

The colour on the plate will also help you get all the vitamins and minerals that we require, which some of us of us are deficient in. Do you want to avoid certain diseases and illnesses? Well, we've got to make sure we are getting vitamins and minerals which we may have missed out on through having processed food.

So we need real food, with real colour, and therefore real energy.

If you get away from too much white on your plate, whether it's potatoes, pasta, rice, or noodles, you'll definitely see the benefits.

Leafy things that grow above the ground, Brussels sprouts, cabbages, cauliflowers, lettuces, are typically really high in nutrients and low in calories.

But potatoes and kumara are the ones that are really energy dense.

Fats aren't always villains

We used to think that all fats were automatically bad. But that's not the case.

A little butter on your steamed green vegetables, some avocado oil on your salad, some good health nuts in your salad, a little good-quality cheese — these things are very good, because they keep you satisfied for longer.

The body requires fat to function. As well as basic body processes, fats are also really important for healthy joints and reduced inflammation.

Fat is very dense in energy and requires a bit more time and effort for the body to process.

Good fats are natural fats: butter, oils from nuts and seeds, flaxseed oil, avocado oil, olive oil, all those good oils that are full of good omegas. Or natural fatty foods such as avocados, nuts and seeds.

All these foods provide good energy for a long period of time. A really good example of this is an experiment I remember doing at school. You get a peanut and you set it on fire. It'll burn for five minutes. If you get a peanut-sized piece of candy floss or cube of sugar and set that on fire, it is gone in 10 seconds.

That's exactly what happens in the body.

The peanut will give us better sustained energy over a longer period of time than that simple carbohydrate, the sugar, which will just go just like that. And then what will happen is that we'll get hungry again.

So at the end of the day we've eaten twice as much food because we had lots of carbohydrates and not enough protein. You'll have peaks and troughs of energy, feel tired and flat, and will want to eat more to feel okay. It becomes a roller coaster.

But if you have lots of healthy fats in your day, those peaks and troughs tend to flatten out. And that's what we're trying to achieve, a constant, level energy through the day, as opposed to a roller-coaster ride.

Round the edge is best

Now, as we set out on the journey of being healthier, it is far easier to eat well if you shop well. The thing I like to do is shop, usually with my daughter, around the edge of the supermarket.

People may have heard that before, but don't understand why. It's really pretty simple. Everything around the edge of the supermarket is refrigerated because it is usually real, whole food, and it needs to be chilled. If it's not chilled it'll go bad, because it tends not to be pumped up with preservatives, additives or chemical colours like the stuff in the aisles.

The food in the aisles is often processed, full of calories, artificial, and disappears quickly in your body to be stored as fat if you don't use it in exercise straight away.

If you shop on the edges of the supermarket, you get your colour, you get your nutrients, and it doesn't cost any more than the food in the aisles. And, talking about cost, when you go down the aisles a lot, you'll run the risk of buying stuff you don't really need.

Do I go down the aisles at all? Yes. But with specific things in mind. Maybe a little bit of chocolate, some coffee, and cleaning things for the house.

Stick mostly to the edges: it's part of the next step to eating well for life.

Make organisation your friend

Take a little time to work out what you're going to need to eat during the week, so you can shop for it.

For example, look at what you might be having for breakfast this week. Maybe some eggs, some avocado, a berry smoothie, and some muesli. Making sure you have a list and buy what you need is shopping well.

You might think about the fact you get hungry at work. If you buy some almonds and some fruit and take them to work, you won't have to buy something from a café, like a sausage roll. Making sure you've got the ability to eat well with what you've brought from home means you don't have to buy something convenient, but unhealthy.

Know what you're buying

I strongly recommend a phone app called 'My Fitness Pal'. (Full disclosure: I have no commercial connection with this app, I just use it and think it's fantastic.)

Basically you type what the food is, and it acts as a calorie counter, but more importantly, it tells you what's actually in your food. With the app you can discover, for example, that a fresh apple has 210 kilojoules (about three teaspoons) of sugar in it, while a glass of orange juice has 500 kilojoules of sugar (about seven teaspoons), and a 30-gram serving of Kellogg's rice bubbles, which is quite a small serve, has about the same amount of sugar. So we can find out which foods have a lot of sugar which, we know, if stored in the body, can convert to fat.

It's becoming clearer, as every year goes by, that there's a need to try to eat real food. Processed food is full of artificial ingredients, additives, preservatives, colours and flavourings. That will change the nutrient profile of that food.

We all need nutrients and vitamins and minerals to function and adapt and recover and grow and learn, and by having artificial food, or food that is full of chemicals, we are probably not getting the nutrients we need, and we are probably ingesting stuff that is not good for us in the long term.

If you look at what is happening in the world in terms of health, there's a greater incidence of major diseases and health issues than there used to be. Yes, we have got a longer lifespan, but we've got more major diseases than we have ever had. Is that because of all the crappy stuff we are chucking in our food? Is it because of the lifestyles we are leading? Or is it somehow all intertwined?

There have been some amazing studies around the world of populations not living in first-world environments whose health is good. Typically their food doesn't contain all the artificial rubbish that we have in ours.

The All Blacks know you can't out-train bad nutrition

People wanting to get fit, and lose weight, will often try to do more exercise but not change how they eat. Or people will try to change how they eat but not worry about doing any exercise.

The fact is, these things have to work hand in hand. The healthiest lifestyle will be one that has regular activity and smart nutrition. It doesn't mean you diet — you don't diet. You get the relationship right between the two, activity and eating, and it's sustainable. Even the All Blacks, as professional athletes, learn pretty quickly that you can't out-train a bad diet.

The good thing is that, if anything, you can improve your ability by improving your diet. A good example is, if you're trying to get quicker, you can do all the speed training in the world, but if you're carrying three extra kilos you're not going to be faster. Sometimes it's easier to lose those three kilos to get quicker by eating better.

Or maybe you're wanting to improve your ability to run 3km in a test that we might do with the All Blacks. You can be training the house down and working really hard but if you then eat poorly afterwards, the benefits you were going to get are undone by what you have just eaten.

Most good athletes now realise you are what you eat. Get your training sorted, which is often the easy part, and then improve your nutrition. Get that perfect, and it's a far, far easier job.

It's very easy to have a great body composition and a great physique if you train hard and eat well — but you can't achieve that without doing both.

If you want a hand getting on top of your health and fitness, get in touch with Gilly. Website: nicgill.com, Instagram: nicgill_health_and_performance

WELSH WISDOM

When Welsh-born Phil Kingsley Jones is not at work as the business manager of the Counties Manukau Rugby Union he's a stand-up comedian, and the author, with Stu Wilson, of a series of bestselling joke books. Here's his joke for blokes.

The head coach of the Thames Valley Roller Mills primary school rugby team is approached by a well-known car dealer who says to the coach, 'I'll give you any car off my yard if you select my boy.'

The coach says, 'I can't do that. It's bribery.'

'Well,' says the dealer, 'give me $20 and you can say you paid for it.'

'Good idea,' the coach says. 'Here's $40. I'll have two.'

Stroke
Dodging the Sniper Fire

Think of a stroke as an enemy sniper during war time. The best course of action with a stroke or a sniper is to avoid being hit at all. Soldiers rely on intelligence reports to warn them where and when a sniper is operating. With a stroke your doctor is the intel expert, who can spot menacing signs, and find ways to counter the danger.

If you are hit with a stroke, then, just as with a wound from a sniper, the faster the treatment the better the recovery. Let's begin with how to avoid the stroke bullet.

Start with prevention, says John Gommans, the chairman of the Stroke Foundation of New Zealand, and the chief medical officer at Hawke's Bay Hospital.

There are two main paths to stroke safety. One is to have your blood pressure checked, and, if there's a problem, getting it under control. The other is smoking. 'Stopping smoking,' says John, 'is more effective than most of the pills I can give you.'

When should you start checking your risk of a stroke?

'In general terms, most men should have a cardiovascular health check in their mid-40s. If there is a family history of strokes, you should start having your blood pressure monitored 10 years earlier. And, if you are Maori, Pacific Islander, or from the Indian sub-continent, you should be having a check-up from the time you're 35.

'Sadly there is an ethnic element with strokes. For Maori and Pasifika people strokes not only come on earlier in life, but they tend to have worse outcomes.'

Your health professional, whether it's a doctor or a nurse, can look for hidden factors that can lead to a stroke. As well as blood pressure, you'll probably be checked for diabetes, cholesterol levels, and any underlying heart conditions, especially an irregular heart rhythm.

Why are these checks so hugely worthwhile?

Because if you have more than one risk factor, the nasty fact about your chance of a stroke is that risk factors don't add up, they multiply. 'So it makes it even more important that you work on all the problems, not just the easy ones,' says Gommans.

What will you be offered if your blood pressure is putting you into stroke territory?

'If diet and exercise aren't enough to control your blood pressure,' says John, 'there's a wide range of medication available, and your doctor will help you decide what's best for you. Remember that once you start using blood pressure-lowering medication you may be on them for life. You should only stop on your doctor's advice.'

If you've already had a stroke, or are at very high risk of having one, you will probably be given some blood-thinning medication. It may be as simple, and old-fashioned, as taking aspirin, a drug that's been around for over 100 years.

Aspirin, says John, is a 'mild blood thinner'. There are also other, newer drugs, which are at least as good as aspirin, and possibly a little better.

If you do suffer a stroke, then realising what's happened, and acting on it, is crucial.

What you need to do, says John, is very simple: 'If you do get symptoms of a stroke then don't muck around, just call the ambulance. Speed is hugely important.'

So if you are having a stroke, what are the vital signs to look for? The Stroke Foundation uses the acronym FAST to help you remember . . .

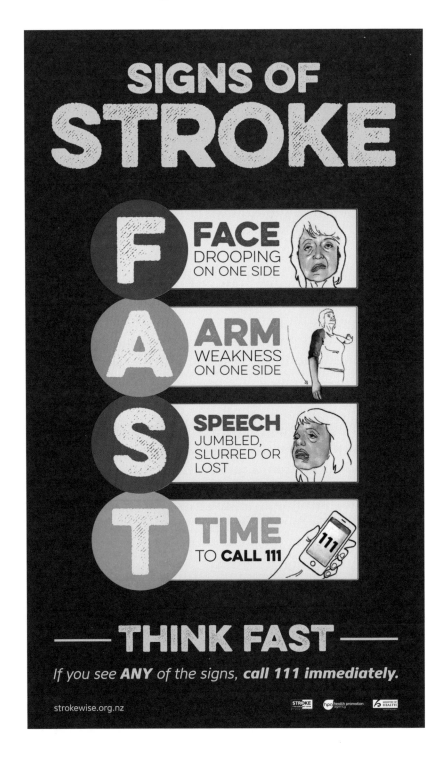

The FAST test will pick up 80% of strokes, but there are other signs. Double vision or blurred vision in one eye, or part of both eyes. A sudden weakness or numbness in one leg. A sudden loss of balance, an unexplained fall, or difficulty controlling movement, especially when they occur with some of the other symptoms.

A stroke is a problem with the blood supply to the brain. 'It can be due to either a blockage in the blood vessels,' says John, 'so the blood stops coming through, or you burst the pipe and the blood leaks out, and therefore doesn't get to a part of the brain.

'So there are two different ways it happens, but the end result is part of the brain doesn't get the blood it needs to live on, and therefore stops working.'

Why is speedy treatment so important?

'One treatment option we have is what is quite often called the clot-busting or clot-dissolving drugs. If we are going to give this to you to make a difference for your stroke, that is best done as soon as possible within the first three, or maybe four, hours, but it is dangerous after four and a half hours.

'We need someone to recognise they are having a stroke, call an ambulance, and get into the hospital in time for us to do the assessments and the scans, and give them the drug, all preferably within three hours.

'The brain, unlike the heart, is very specialised. Different parts of the brain do very different things. So what happens with your particular stroke depends on which blood vessel happens to be damaged or blocked.'

If you think of a man with a stroke as someone who drags a leg when he walks, or has an arm that won't work, they are classic effects of a stroke. But not the only ones.

'If the blood vessel that's blocked or damaged is the one that feeds the part of the brain that controls movement on one side of the body, then you have a problem with that.

'And that is the most common. But there are other parts of the brain, of course, involved in memory, speech, emotions, vision, thinking and balance. You can't easily compare one person's stroke with another, they are all a bit individual.'

How much do strokes vary in intensity?

'If you block a big blood vessel that feeds a big part of your brain you are going to have a lot of damage to your brain, so you have more disability and much less chance of recovery.

'On the other hand, if you're lucky and you have a very small clot and it blocks a very small blood vessel that is feeding a tiny part of the brain, you can completely recover, or even have such a mild stroke while you sleep you don't even know you have had it.

'We can do a brain scan and see what we call silent strokes. People often have had two or three earlier strokes that they don't even know they have had.

'Another thing is what we often call the mini-strokes. The technical term is TIA, which stands for a transient (as in temporary), ischaemic (a Greek word for lack of blood supply) attack.

If a clot blocks a blood vessel, and your brain stops working for a short time, your body can sometimes dissolve the clot by itself. If the blood supply comes back before any permanent damage is done, you can have a full recovery. And that is what we call a mini-stroke.

'So people start speaking in a funny way or are paralysed in an arm and a leg for 10 or 20 minutes or so, and then fully recover. They think, "Oh, it's fully recovered, I don't need to worry about that."

'But what we know is a lot of those mini-strokes are rapidly followed by a major stroke. However, if we get in early after a TIA and give drugs to thin the blood a bit, and control the blood pressure, and look at cholesterol, and help you to stop smoking, we can dramatically cut your risk of going on to have that big follow-up stroke.

'Think of a TIA as a warning shot above your head. No lasting damage, but time to take action, and to take it fast!'

If you have a massive stroke the harsh reality is that you will probably be left living with disabilities.

On the other hand, strokes are understood a lot better now, and in all reasonably sized hospitals in New Zealand there are specialist stroke units.

'We understand the benefits of being managed by a team of people who know about strokes,' says John Gommans. 'We talk about the importance of being in a stroke unit where you have skilled doctors and nurses.

'Firstly, we reduce your risk of complications. Secondly, we improve the chances of you getting home and living independently, or with lower levels of support required. Thirdly, we also investigate why you had your stroke and what treatments you need to prevent a future stroke.

'With a small stroke, you have a lot more normal, undamaged brain to help compensate while you're learning new ways of doing something.

'We get many more people living at home now than we used to. It's all about trying to improve your quality of life, even if you have got some disability afterwards.'

The Stroke Foundation of New Zealand's website is a mine of information. You'll find it at <u>stroke.org.nz.</u>

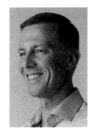

Mark Corbitt

Mark Corbitt came to New Zealand from England with his parents when he was three years old. For most of his life he's lived and worked in Wellington, where he's now the General Manager of Information and Community Technology at Contact Energy. Mark and his wife Susie have a combined family of five children, and are now grandparents for the first time. For a fit and active person, Mark's stroke, in 2015 when he was 50, came out of the blue.

I was on a plane from Sydney to Wellington. About halfway through the flight I had a five-minute incident, and then a long one that lasted the remainder of the flight, which I think by that stage was about another hour and a half, maybe an hour and three-quarters.

I was locked in my seat unable to move, because the left side of my body had classic stroke symptoms. Face drooping, speech slurred and not understandable, and no ability to move the left side of my body at all for the remainder of the flight, and for about another hour afterwards, I guess. I couldn't honestly tell you an exact time because I wasn't really able to do anything.

Who worked out it was a stroke?

I kind of figured it out myself after the short one. I thought, 'This is not right.' Having known some of the basics of a stroke, especially the loss of a side of the body, I kind of guessed that's what it was.

My knowledge basically came from general publicity. I'd seen the FAST (Face, Arms, Speech, Time) acronym before. Frankly, it hadn't had a whole heap of meaning to me until it happened.

When the second one, the major one, occurred, I was cognitively still aware of what was going on, even if physically I couldn't do anything. Believe me, that is one of the worst sensations. I never want to experience that again.

I was medevaced off the flight into Wellington Hospital's emergency department. The speed with which I was able to be treated with emergency blood-thinning treatment was, I believe, a big component in my recovery. They got in and gave me the treatment inside what I understand is a three- to four-hour window when it's effective. Over the next 18 hours I had something like 13 strokes, and then I spent a week in hospital.

I went back to work pretty quickly and, in retrospect, too early. I had a lingering weakness in the left side particularly. I couldn't walk as well as I had been able to previously.

The change in how I walked was almost unnoticeable but I knew that if I wanted to step down stairs, or step up stairs, I had to take extra care. Early on, I got incredibly tired incredibly quickly and just wasn't able to think as fast. It's maybe a weird way of putting it, but it was kind of like being permanently drunk, if that makes sense.

Probably two weeks before the stroke I had had a very minor incident which I took as a blackout, but it turns out it was the first noticeable precursor. It's almost impossible to pinpoint, but I'm told I'd probably been having precursor things, just tiredness or brief gaps, for maybe a year beforehand.

They were probably masked by the fact I was very, very fit. A couple of months before the stroke I'd completed a 100km road cycle ride around Blenheim and Marlborough, the GrapeRide. I'd been fit for 20-odd years. It certainly helped with the recovery, but may well have masked earlier symptoms.

At work, they put us through a full three-hour medical assessment every couple of years, and I'd had one the year before my stroke, and came out in excellent health. I wasn't overweight; maybe a couple of kilos. The assessment came complete with an ECG, a treadmill test, all the blood tests — PSA (prostate) and all that wonderful stuff — and they all came out fine.

But I did have an elevated cholesterol count at the time. Not hugely elevated but enough to be concerned about, which I immediately did something about. I didn't take any pills. It was primarily a change of diet. I halved my sugar intake and salt intake, but I didn't stop eating dairy or animal fats. I was a big cheese eater, a big meat eater. Had been for my entire life; it was the way I was brought up.

That slightly elevated cholesterol level was really the only abnormal factor. That was the only factor that, in retrospect, may have been a warning.

Since the stroke, I've changed my diet a lot. We now eat basically plant-based and whole foods. No dairy, no animal fats.

The only animal, if you will, that I do eat occasionally is fish but, other than that, it's completely plant-based and whole foods and that's made a massive difference to my cholesterol. I'm running at the moment at about 2.7, 2.8 as a cholesterol ratio, and they say that if you're below 3.8 your chance of a stroke and heart disease is pretty minimal.

In general, I feel like I'm better than I was before. The only real residual thing I'm left with is that I have a slightly different sensation in the tips of the fingers on my left hand and sometimes in the sole of my left foot. I haven't had any loss of sensation, it's just the fingers feel things differently than the tips on my right hand. Quite why that is, I've no idea.

But apart from that I'm fitter than I was before. I'm training for the 160km around Taupo cycle ride at the moment.

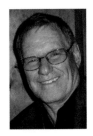

Colin McKenzie

Colin McKenzie started his working life in hotels, but a love of sport, especially rugby league, saw him working in radio, at first in his hometown of Christchurch, and then in Wellington. He toured with the Kiwis in Britain from 1982 into the 1990s, providing news reports and live commentaries. Late in 1995 he and his wife, Lorraine, moved back to Christchurch. In February of 1996 he suffered a stroke. Sadly he wasn't treated with the speed that's needed for a better recovery. Being a sports reporter, always busy in the weekend, Monday was usually his day off. He now calls what happened to him 'running out of Mondays'.

We'd been in Wellington for 10 years and, although the job treated me well, coming home was always the aim. We owned a section in Christchurch and were planning to build.

I was working in the Christchurch newsroom at ZB in 1996. I'd had some blood pressure problems years before that but I thought that was all behind me. I knew best. As long as I hopped on the scales and they told me what I wanted to see, and I could go for a run and a swim, I thought things were fine.

My wife Lorraine was still in Wellington, selling the house and finishing her teaching year, and then she was coming down. I was staying with my mum at her place.

In February 1996 I was on a day off, and I went down to the section. I pulled out a couple of tree roots by hand, and then went for a jog on the beach, very, very quietly. Just a very old man's jog along the beach.

I felt fine until I got to the soft sand heading back to the car in the carpark and my right arm and right leg started feeling a bit limp.

I thought, 'This doesn't feel right.' So I went back home to my mum's and said, 'Could you ring a doctor?' I couldn't hold the paper to read *The Press*, and she thought it might be a stroke. So I just hopped in the car and drove down to the doctor, as you do.

I went into the doctor's at North New Brighton. I hadn't been there in years. I told them at the desk what was wrong and they sent me through to the doctor, and he ran a few tests and said, 'Your blood pressure is dangerously high. Take a Disprin a day and come back on Tuesday.' I think that was on a Thursday. In hindsight, I cursed the man for not taking action immediately.

So I went back out to the desk, arranged Tuesday's appointment and then froze on the spot; I couldn't move. That was the stroke. There was no pain. Just the leg and right arm were even heavier than they had been at the beach, and I couldn't move. I ended up spending nine weeks in hospital where I was treated very, very well indeed.

On the second day, the Mad Butcher arrived. He'd flown down as soon as he heard. Brought all sorts of stuff from the Warriors players and all sorts of messages, it was delightful. Typical Peter Leitch.

From then on a lot of people arrived. People like (Kiwi) Brent Todd, (Kiwi coach) Tank Gordon, are just two off the top of my head. I said, 'How did you know I was here?' Both of them said the same: 'The Butcher told me.'

When I got out of hospital I was told that my right arm would only be a support arm, and I'd have a limp on my right leg, which was held in a calliper.

After a stroke, you've just got to go with the flow. If you've got a lame arm, and find it difficult picking things up, forcing it up will not make any difference.

My right arm has now got a permanent curve in it because I thought I knew better. I got little weights and tried to lift them, and I'd say, 'Come on' and grip and grip and force my arm up. But, for every exercise you do one way with an arm, you've got to do it the other way to relax the muscle again. I was so intent on trying to lift and lift and lift that my arm is more or less permanently bent.

So you've got to do the exercise programme exactly as you're told. There's a reason for it.

After a stroke don't feel bad if you tire quickly, that's just part of it. You may be stuffed halfway through a day, and if you are, you've got to have a rest. You just can't suddenly start leaping around and run around the block.

You've got to be fair when you get home too. Your wife or your partner has got to go on with a certain amount of their life. You can get frustrated when you first go home. You aren't the only concern in the house. You just can't ring a buzzer and get someone to come and do something for you.

Initially, improvements after a stroke usually come fairly quickly. But for me, after that there were no more improvements. Nowadays they'd get you into treatment quickly. They can make big changes now. They can bring about marvellous changes. I had my stroke 20 years ago, so things have changed now.

Living with a stroke, you've got to be aware that your emotions are very close to the surface. You laugh louder, but you're close to tears more quickly. The highs are higher and the lows are lower.

I'm luckier than many as far as speech goes. My speech is not up to broadcast standard, but for normal day-to-day life I can speak quite well.

Walking is a bit of an effort, but I still walk around home. I've got a loop, up and down the drive then around the house, and I pick up the leaves when I'm going. We've got a quarter-acre section and that's my daily walk.

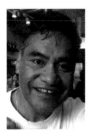

Mau Moananu

Eight years ago, when he was 41, Mau Moananu was working as a manager at Work and Income in Wellington, where he'd been for about 20 years. He had some health issues, but didn't really take them seriously. Then he had a stroke.

Before my stroke, I would eat too much, I would drink, I smoked. I guess you could call it abuse of the human body. The way that I lived then, I was always up until late at night and I was gone early in the morning. I slept very little.

I didn't have any major illnesses but I did have regular visits to the doctor, and he told me that I needed to take pills for high blood pressure. I'd say, 'Oh yeah, yeah, yeah, sweet as, sweet as.'

Then I'd take the pills for about a month. But when they ran out, instead of going back and getting more, I wouldn't go back for three months, six months.

This went on for two or three years. My doctor is really good. He wasn't the problem. The trouble was I felt I was Superman, you know.

My stroke happened at my home. When I woke up that morning I went to go to the loo, as normal. But, when I got up, I started sort of limping on my right side on the way down to the toilet. I thought, 'Oh, it must be some pins and needles.'

When I went back to my bedroom, I said to myself, 'I'll just sit here on the bed for a little while.' But my right side was getting more and more paralysed.

And then I tried to talk to my son, and all that came out was some sort of strange language. I was getting angry because I was thinking they should understand what I'm saying, but it was getting worse and worse. I got up and I tried to get changed into my work clothes, but I was struggling to get my pants on.

It was my sister who recognised that it was a stroke. She's worked in Wellington Hospital for many years, and was always up to date with these sorts of things. When I was trying to talk, to communicate with her, she said, 'Oh my gosh, you're having a stroke' or something like that. She called an ambulance.

The ambulance came straight away, and I remember them giving something to me, because I was getting less and less able to move. They told me to just lie down, and I'm pretty sure they gave me something with a needle. My memory starts to falter a bit there, because I was starting to black out.

I was in hospital for about nine or ten weeks. For the first four or five weeks, I couldn't move my right side at all, and I think there was a chance I was going to die. A lot of people were coming to see me, but I wasn't aware of much in those first few weeks.

My recovery began at the hospital. They had speech therapists, and they had physios to help me get better. But there was only so much they could do after that, because when they released me I was released, of course, back into normal life.

About a month after the stroke, my kids were crying for me, and that was the day I decided I was going to make a better life for myself, and for all those around me.

I started going to the gym; I started going for walks; I started watching what I ate, and I gave up smoking. I dropped my drinking right down. I lost a lot of weight.

I had to look and see what had been wrong with me, and why it had happened. From there my aim was to make it better. If I'd always lived the way I do now I would have cut my risk of a stroke right down, maybe to zero.

I still take some pills. I take them religiously, but there's been a drastic reduction in the number over time. I take some to keep my cholesterol levels down, to control my blood pressure, and another for my heart. Now my doctor says my health is better than it was 20 years ago.

I've still only got 55% function on my right side, but I'm able to do a lot of things. In February 2016, I was in a group on a nationwide bike ride to raise awareness of Maori and Pasifika health, and I was able to ride 720km.

I was able to go back to work (at Work and Income). I was there for three more years but, in reality, it wasn't the job for me any more. I had six months off with no job.

Then I found a job with IHC helping people who are intellectually disabled. I look after people from five-year-olds up to 75-year-olds, and it was what I was looking for. I find the work really satisfying.

JEREMY CORBETT'S HEALTH STORY

Jeremy Corbett is the host of the long-running comedy show 7 Days *on TV3. He has also fronted an award-winning breakfast show on More FM. Health is a concern for him, and he admits that in recent years he and his wife have gained 30kg: 'Apparently they're called kids.'*

I'm such a believer in the prostate check that whenever I see my doctor I demand he get the glove on and have a 'look around'.

He's usually reluctant and says things like, 'This isn't a consultation, we're only playing golf.'

But I insist. Better safe than sorry.

Those golf gloves are not as comfortable as a surgical glove though.

Skin Cancer
The Spots and Specks

Aussies will always be our great rivals. When we beat them at rugby, league, netball, basketball or football, we love it. And no wonder.

I once walked into a toilet during a rugby test in Sydney to find a local had written on the wall above a urinal, 'In Australia we wash our hands after we've been to the dunny.'

Someone, obviously a Kiwi, had written underneath, 'In New Zealand they teach us not to pee on our hands.'

However, there's one field, skin cancer rates, especially melanoma, where, to be honest, they do a lot better than us. There are various reasons why the guys from across the ditch lead the way when it comes to limiting the amount of damage done by skin cancers.

One's just our bad luck. The ultraviolet rays that trigger skin cancer kick in at much lower temperatures here. We live in a beautiful country, but our sun can literally be a killer.

To be fair, another is that the Aussies started off 'slip, slop, slap' campaigns for skin protection back in the 1980s, much earlier than we did.

So what can be done to make things better here? Let's start with age.

Sadly, if kids aren't covered up with hats, clothes and sunscreen, then 80% of the damage to their skin has been done by the time they're 20.

It doesn't have to be that way. Right now, if you're a dad, or a grandad, there's a massive role for you in helping to prevent your kids, or grandkids, from getting skin cancer.

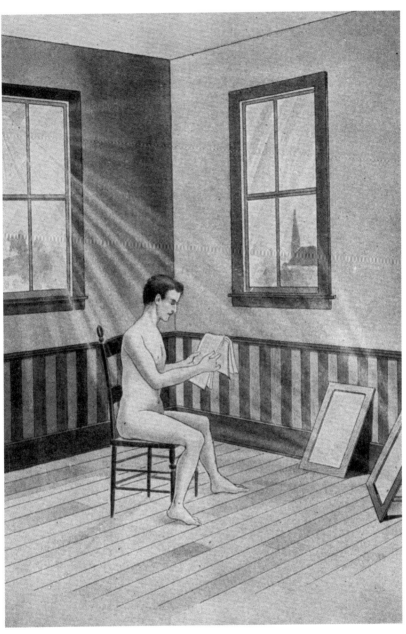

In an English health manual from 1924, indoor sunbathing, with mirrors aiding the process, was said to 'restore the feeble and invigorate the debilitated' better than any drug remedy. No mention then of 'slip, slop, slap'.

At the beach, or even just playing outside, there are good rash suits that block UV rays. Add a hat and you've potentially lifeguarded a child you love. Cover from clothing designed to screen out UV rays is the best protection.

There will be times, playing cricket for example, when a kid's arms can't really be covered. Sunscreen is the answer there, but remember to keep reapplying the sunscreen every couple of hours.

Experts also say it's vital to check out the use-by date on sunscreen. If the sunscreen is past its expiry date, a child may look protected, but he or she is at risk.

If you're in your 20s, 30s or 40s, hopefully you treat yourself in the sun the same way kids should be looked after. But let's say you're a bit older, and grew up when the aim in summer was to try to get brown, even if, like me, most of your ancestors were from Scotland and Northern Ireland, and you had pale, easily burnt skin. You might have been from an era when instead of sunscreen, you slapped on coconut oil, so your skin sizzled and fried under the summer sun.

Dr Anthony Tam, a dermatoscopist, a dermatologic surgeon and a clinical advisor to the charitable trust Melanoma New Zealand (in other words an expert on the detection and treatment of skin cancer), offers informed advice.

'If you are at risk, what you should do is get yourself along to a medical person and have an all-over, once-over check. Even if it is just once, get it done by someone who knows what they're doing.'

There are three main forms of skin cancer: melanoma, squamous cell cancers, and basal cell cancers.

'To put things into perspective,' says Anthony, 'there are around 490 deaths in New Zealand from skin cancer each year. Approximately 360 of those are from melanoma, so that is why it gets all the attention.

'Of the remainder, most of those are squamous cell cancers that cause death. You will see figures saying one in three people in New Zealand will get skin cancer. That mostly relates to the less aggressive basal cell cancers.

'A recent New Zealand study canvassed a whole range of people and it was surprising that in the older age bracket, many thought melanoma was a disease of younger people. In actual fact, it is the older age bracket who suffer the most, and it is more lethal in older guys. It is just that when it hits younger people, there can be young families involved, and the sufferers are often in the prime of their lives, so it is often perceived in a diffcrent light.'

Where should you begin to make sure you're not one of the statistics?

Anthony suggests being checked if you or your partner is concerned about any growths on your skin. 'I had someone recently and he only had his melanoma diagnosed because his wife was peotoring him about something on his back. So listen to others, just get it looked at once, even just for peace of mind, and then go from there.'

You can start with your doctor, who may decide to send you to a skin cancer specialist.

What will the examination involve?

Before you go, remember to follow the advice your mum used to give you years ago: wear clean undies when you went out in case you had a car accident. Because for the examination you'll be asked to undress to your underwear while the specialist examines your skin.

He, or she, will use a dermatoscope, a device Anthony says is 'like a stethoscope for the skin. It's like a magnifying glass, but it helps us to see through the skin more than a normal magnifying glass would. You can work out what's a melanoma, and what's just a mole.

'It takes a lot of training and experience, but once you're there you're six times as accurate in picking up melanoma.'

Keep in mind skin cancer can develop anywhere there's skin. Anthony says he tells his patients he will examine every inch of their body if they have any concerns. It's rare, but he has removed skin cancer from the head of a penis.

Hopefully the examination will show you're clear. In itself, that's a boost to how you feel.

'In terms of empowerment,' says Anthony, 'often when people walk out they will say, "Look, that's a tremendous relief, I'm going to keep coming back just so I know that this is what I can do to enjoy life." You've got to a certain level; why not do everything in your power to make sure you stay healthy?'

If something dubious is found, you'll be called back for a biopsy under local anaesthetic.

Under sterile conditions the skin will be injected to numb it. There'll be a 2-millimetre margin marked out around the affected area, or lesion. That area will be cut out as an ellipse (the shape of a rugby ball) so the skin will later come together neatly when it's stitched.

What's been cut out is sent to a lab. 'If the lab says it's fine, then you carry on,' says Anthony.

How much treatment is needed for melanoma depends on how deep it is. If it is what's called melanoma in situ, and hasn't invaded through the epidermal membrane (a layer between your skin and the other tissues in your body), the chance of a full recovery is virtually 100%.

If it's undetected and metastasises (and spreads through the rest of your body, which is also known as stage 4), the chances of recovery are dramatically worse.

In plain terms, if a melanoma is found when it's less than a millimetre thick go to the bank that in five years' time it won't have endangered your life. Sadly, if it's 4 millimetres or more thick, and it's ulcerated, there's only a four in 10 chance you'll survive the next five years.

How to beat the odds?

Cover up when you're young, so skin cancer doesn't even get a start. And, if it's too late for that, then early detection is the key. Find a skin cancer early, and there's every chance you'll fare as well as those sun-smart Aussies.

The Cancer Society of New Zealand has a highly detailed online booklet on melanoma. Go to their website, cancernz.org.nz, click on 'cancer information', then on 'cancer types', and then on 'melanoma'. You'll see the downloadable PDF booklet on the right of the screen.

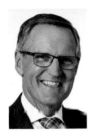

Peter Williams

Peter Williams is a household name and face. He's been a television reporter and presenter at TVNZ for 30 years, covering rugby, cricket and eight Olympic Games, including the latest Games in Rio. He's also been a newsreader, and a host of Mastermind. A private man away from the cameras, he's stayed fit and largely healthy. But, over time, the endless summers of his youth have caught up with him in the form of skin cancers.

I was living in Wellington. It was around about 1992. A little scab on my lip just wouldn't clear up, so I went to the doctor about it, and he advised that it was basal cell carcinoma and it needed a plastic surgeon to remove it.

So I dutifully went off to a clinic somewhere in Lower Hutt. It was a procedure that only lasted about 20 minutes, maybe half an hour. I got a jab in the lip and had a mask put over my face and this thing was nicked out. There was a stitch in it for a few days but then it was fine, and that was that.

About 10 years later another one of these things showed up on my lip, and I went to the doctor, who put me in touch with a plastic surgeon again.

This time it was called a squamous cell carcinoma, an SCC, which is a little bit more serious. They can develop into full-blown, real problem-causing cancers, so that was also nicked out with a similar procedure.

It was at a clinic in Remuera. Cary Mellow, who is a top plastic surgeon in Auckland, did the job, and again it was a relatively short procedure. Took 15, 20 minutes. You get a jab in the lip, you drive yourself home that night, there's a stitch there and it clears itself up.

That one was a wee bit bigger, and left a longer scar. In fact, I've still got the scar on my face to this day down the side of my lip on the left-hand side.

Never thought too much about skin cancer after that, but my wife would say to me every now and then when she saw me with my shirt off, 'Gosh, that doesn't look too good.'

I'd have them examined by a doctor every now and then, but it was really when I stayed at the hotel in Melbourne, during the Cricket World Cup final in March 2015, that I really started to pay attention to what was going on.

The configuration of the hotel room was such that there was a mirror on each wall. So when you looked at yourself in the mirror to do your hair, there was a mirror behind, and I could see my back, and I was bloody horrified by what I saw.

You never look at your back, but I saw this big black spot on my shoulder blades. I thought, 'Hell, that just doesn't look very good at all.'

So off I went to the GP who referred me to one of his colleagues who is a skin specialist, and that was diagnosed through a biopsy as a melanoma in situ which means that it's potentially in the surface on your skin and hasn't permeated into the rest of your body. He also looked at some other little spots and the like on my face, and on my back, and found there were about three or four other basal cell carcinomas.

So over the course of 2015, I had about half a dozen of these things removed. Two or three sessions down at the GP's clinic, CityMed down in Albert Street.

Each of the sessions lasted about an hour or so. You get a local anaesthetic and it's nicked out. It's not particularly uncomfortable. The only really uncomfortable part is when they're stitching you back together again and they're pulling the skin.

The last procedure I had was after getting back from the Rugby World Cup in November 2015. I had a BCC removed from my forehead just below the hairline, so again Cary Mellow did that.

There were one or two other little spots that you can now clear up with a cream, a fairly high-octane cream that you apply at night when you go to bed, about five times a week for about six weeks. It blows up into a horrible bloody scab and then, once the scab falls off, the basal cell carcinoma, or the skin damage, is cleared up.

The last couple of years I have spent too much time having this stuff removed, but I think it's for the greater good. There's no doubt that the problems I've had date back to my schooldays when getting tanned was a badge of honour.

We lived in Invercargill when I was at primary school, and the summer sun is really harsh there. I got sunburned so badly once I had blisters on each shoulder. I can clearly remember this. The blisters were the size of half a golf ball. They were really big suckers, and so that was pretty bad.

I spent a summer between my sixth- and seventh-form years working as a labourer in a forest, just south of Oamaru, trimming trees and debarking wood, and that sort of thing. Good physical work. Hot as hell and every time the sun came out we took the shirt off, and got ourselves a suntan with no sun cream at all. I had a great suntan, I was the envy of all my mates because of all the outdoor work I was doing. But it certainly hasn't been very rewarding 45 years on.

These days I wouldn't be seen dead with my shirt off anywhere, apart from an indoor swimming pool. Even when I go swimming at Parnell at the saltwater baths I always put a wetsuit on. I'd never go swimming in togs any more. I'm absolutely dead-set scared of being outside and being exposed.

Of course the other thing when I was younger, I played a lot of golf, a lot of cricket, and you never wore hats in those days or put cream on any part of your ears or nose.

During the heat of the summer you've got to make sure that you spray yourself, and lather particularly your ears, and your nose, and around the back of your neck. I always like to play golf with my collar up to make sure I'm not affected.

It's quite extraordinary the number of old golf pros, guys in their 60s now, who have got the tops of their ears nicked off because even though they might have worn caps in the day, they had their ears exposed and, later on, they've had little skin cancers on the tops of their ears.

ROAD REST . . .

Dai Henwood is a Billy T James award-winning comedian, a team leader on the show 7 Days, *and the frontman on TV3's* Family Feud. *He has what almost amounts to a fetish for orange road cones, and roadworks.*

I see a lot of road workers resting, and it makes me wonder why they are not called road resters.

Doing some investigation, I saw a group of road workers being spoken to by the Chief Road Worker (I think that is the correct term).

I walked up to listen to what the chief was saying and it didn't surprise me . . .

'Okay crew, the trucks are running a bit late so, it would be great if you can lean on each other until the shovels arrive.'

Smoking
Stubbing Out the Habit

Don't ever feel bad about finding it hard to give up smoking. You're kicking the most sophisticated, crafty addiction in the world, one designed that way by the best scientific minds big tobacco money can buy.

But if you do quit, the benefits to your health will be bigger than Donald Trump's ego.

To be specific, let's take an example. You're 45 and have been smoking for more than 25 years. Your risk of a heart attack is three times greater than a 45-year-old who's never smoked.

When you stop smoking, no matter how old you are, here are the great things that happen. After 12 hours your blood oxygen level will be back to that of a non-smoker. After 48 hours damaged nerve endings start to regrow. After two weeks your heart attack risk starts to decline. After a year your risk of a heart attack or stroke has halved. So the benefits are enormous.

I won't insult your intelligence by saying quitting will be easy. You might be lucky enough to be one of the handful of people, with low addiction genes, who overnight smokes a last cigarette, throws the pack in the rubbish and never smokes again.

The odds are, you won't be. But never feel bad about how many times it takes you to stop.

Boyd Broughton, a health promoter from ASH (Action on Smoking and Health New Zealand), says the average smoker has 12 attempts before finally stopping.

On the upside of the statistics, stop smoking for a month, that's ONE month, and it's almost certain you will never smoke again.

The addictive drug you're fighting is nicotine, which occurs naturally in tobacco leaves. Your brain reacts to nicotine in much the same way as it does to heroin or cocaine. A chemical called dopamine is triggered, and released in your brain. What happens inside your brain then is extremely complex, but the results are pretty straightforward. Basically, you feel good.

Draw on a cigarette and within 10 seconds the high from dopamine's effects is kicking in. Tragically, to get that high you're poisoning yourself, literally speeding up the process of dying.

How bad is smoking for your health?

Smoking contributes to a massive range of fatal diseases. America's government-funded National Cancer Institute says smoking is the single greatest cause of premature and preventable death. Of the deaths directly related to smoking 39% come from heart attacks and strokes, 36% from cancer and 24% from lung disease. In Britain, Cancer Research UK says 86% of lung cancer is caused by smoking.

Trying to put a pretty face on smoking is impossible. As Barack Obama famously said in 2008, 'You can put lipstick on a pig. It's still a pig.'

There are products that kill people, like cars and guns and knives and alcohol and even, if you drink enough of them, sugary soft drinks. But cars, guns, knives, alcohol and soft drinks, when used correctly, don't kill people. When cigarettes are used correctly they still kill people.

America's National Cancer Institute says 250 chemicals have been detected in cigarettes. Of that number, 69 are cancer inducing.

Why so many additives? Because they're needed in cigarettes to not only hide the poison hidden within, but also to make the process of smoking as pleasant an experience as possible.

'A cigarette is a finely crafted nicotine delivery system, and scientists have built it and designed it specially to get that nicotine to your brain,' says Boyd Broughton. 'Normally when you burn something it just ignites and burns really quickly. So they have got chemicals to make sure it doesn't burn too quickly. And they have chemicals that make it taste sweeter. They add different flavours to make it taste sweeter, they have menthol, they do whatever they can to make it attractive.'

Weirdly, nicotine itself isn't harmful. But it plays a huge role in the damage cigarettes do. It's the part of a smoke that makes you a tobacco junkie, the Devil inside the Trojan horse that gets you hooked. Then it's the additives that do the damage.

As with many drugs, the deadly catch-22 with nicotine is that the more you use it, the less effective it becomes.

It's what makes nicotine drug dealers (we could call them cigarette makers but that makes them sound respectable) so staggeringly, Scrooge McDuck money bin, disgustingly, filthy rich.

Once smoking gets its hooks in, only more smoking satisfies the cravings. If you're a long-term smoker have you ever noticed how great the first smoke of the day feels. Why? Because even overnight your dopamine levels have dropped, and the first smoke of the day tops them up. The trouble is, as you probably know, every day that goes by you need to smoke more and more to get the same effect.

So what's the best way to fight an addiction that revolves around a designer drug?

The first step is to want to stop, and it'll probably help to clearly work out your motives. You might only need one reason. There are plenty to choose from. There are the huge benefits to your own health. Heart attacks, strokes, lung diseases and cancer — all less likely if you're not smoking. There are the savings you'll make. Around $16 of tax comes out of your pocket with every pack of cigarettes bought, and the plan is for them to become more expensive with the passing years.

Or it might be the feel-good factor, of setting an example for your own children or grandchildren. Kids are influenced more by example than by words. And, let's be honest, a packet of cigarettes on the kitchen bench, or in the car, even if you never smoke inside the house, or while they're travelling with you, makes smoking look like something normal or even desirable.

(In passing, one great bit of news is that smoking is becoming less and less cool amongst kids. There are huge government surveys of about 30,000 Kiwi schoolchildren each year and the latest shows that 97% of Year 10 Kiwi schoolkids, aged between 13 and 15, don't smoke. Given that the average age for starting to smoke is 12, which drops to even younger children in the case of Maori, the signs look good for future generations to be smoke free.)

Heroes come in various forms. If you've smoked for years, stopping will not only give you a better chance for a long and healthy life, but you'll also be saving your kids, or grandkids, from the illness and misery that long-term smoking causes.

Whatever your motive, once your aim is to stop, says Boyd Broughton, 'You have to have a plan in place.'

Because nicotine addiction is so strong, seek out whatever can help you. Your doctor is a good place to start. If he or she isn't extremely supportive, get a new GP. You're doing yourself and your family and your doctor a big favour by quitting. You can ease cravings for nicotine with various aids such as nicotine patches, gum, or lozenges. It's important, says Boyd, to recognise what the aids do, and also what they can't do.

'People need to know that the patches, gum and lozenges aren't magic,' he says. 'All they do is give you nicotine. It's not as fast as a cigarette, which gets the nicotine to your brain in a matter of seconds, with a really quick hit.'

Don't panic if the alternative ways take longer to kick in.

'The gum is quite quick, while the lozenges are about as quick as the gum. So in maybe five to 10 minutes you get nicotine. There are inhalers now, and they're quite quick too. Patches take longer. After about half an hour it builds the nicotine into your system. But all the technology that we have to get the nicotine to people safely is still slower than a cigarette.'

When you're making your cunning plan to outwit the tobacco

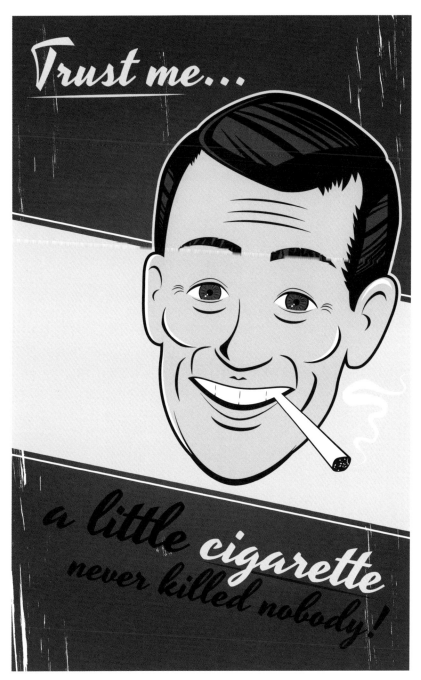

It's true what they said in the good old days. Smoking never killed nobody.
On the other hand, it killed millions of somebodies.

barons, another good idea is to take a look at when you smoke, and what triggers the urge.

'A lot of people say, "I only smoke when I drink, and I don't want to stop drinking",' says Boyd. 'I say, "If you are really serious about stopping smoking, I don't want you to give up drinking forever, in moderation. But this first month is the real challenge, the hardest part to get through. If you can get over the first month without smoking a single cigarette, you have a really good chance of staying smoke free for the rest of your life."

'So when they ask me about the drinking, I say, "If you're really serious about stopping smoking, just for this first month, give up the alcohol. If you're going out drinking, let your friends know what you're trying to achieve. I guarantee there won't be a single mate who will want you to carry on smoking."'

Take a little time to plan ahead and think about what barriers there may be to your goal. As one example, when you go out, don't get a table outside where smoking may be allowed. Look for an inside table.

The great thing today is that you will have universal support for quitting. It hasn't always been so. In the 1970s in New Zealand, when tobacco companies sponsored a lot of sports, threats of banning cigarette sponsorship were greeted with screams of horror from the tobacco companies and their supporters. Sport as we knew it, they claimed, was doomed if the do-gooders had their way. Sport, of course, carried on perfectly well.

Tobacco companies now take a slightly different tack, which is that everyone knows that smoking is bad for you, so if you, as an adult, choose to smoke, that's your informed choice. Which would be a logical argument if research didn't show that most people first try smoking at the age of 12.

Boyd Broughton worries that while it's true most people know that smoking is bad, many don't realise how bad it is also for their loved ones, who don't smoke, and especially for their children.

'There are always exceptions to everything. There may be a great-grandad who smoked, and lived until he was 90. But I'm pretty sure if he thought about it, he wouldn't want his beautiful little grandchildren or great-grandchildren to smoke a cigarette. So it's not just the physical harm you do to yourself when you smoke, but the example being set, which may harm the younger generations.'

If you're quitting smoking, hang in there if you can. In 1964, when I was 17, my father, who had smoked heavily since he'd left school, died of a heart attack after suffering for years from emphysema, a vicious lung disease that can make it almost impossible to breathe.

He'd been a dairy farmer, strong and practical, able to turn his hand from hammering in a fence strainer to changing a wheel on a Farmall tractor, or lifting milk cans into the tray of the farm truck.

By the time he was in his mid-50s, in the grip of emphysema, walking 100 metres to the gate from the farm cottage we lived in near Waihi was a marathon.

There were two urgent calls to his hospital bedside when they thought he was dying. In my last year of high school I was woken by my mother screaming in the early hours of the morning. Dad was on his hands and knees beside their bed, trying desperately to clear the foam that had risen out of his lungs and was choking him.

He was a warm, kind man. I saw at first hand how much he loved his first grandchild, Simon. When he died he was just 59.

Every year that I've lived past his age I've hated how cigarettes, which when he started were still promoted by doctors and sportspeople, robbed him of what should have been years as a doting grandfather.

I hope you understand why, when I say every possible good wish with stopping your smoking, I've never meant anything more.

For good advice, and ways to help you quit, Smokefree New Zealand's website is http://www.smokefree.org.nz.

The Ministry of Health also has sound information at health.govt.nz/your-health/healthy-living/addictions/smoking.

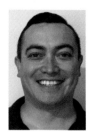

Bern Hoani

Bern Hoani was brought up in Kaikohe in the Far North. In the 1990s, at Northland College, he was a sprinter, a finalist in the national secondary schools' championships, and playing for Northland in rugby and touch. Just before he turned 18, he joined the Army with a handful of mates in 1996. 'There wasn't much for us to do in Kaikohe besides getting into mischief.' In the Army, he concentrated on his academic work and, within three years of leaving in 2000, he was working in IT for major firms such as Telecom and Mainfreight. He now runs an IT business in Melbourne, contracting in Australia and New Zealand, 'punching above our weight with the help of a great team'.

For a person to have quit smoking is a happy-ever-after in my book. I've quit smoking three times. This time it's been five years since I was a slave to the filthy habit.

The habit for me started through a bad association of smoking with comfort. It was my go-to thing when I was stressed. Unbeknown to me at the time, the comfort was actually the action of taking a break, stopping working, taking a moment to gather my thoughts before carrying on with whatever stressful situation I was experiencing.

Smoking while having that break was my downfall, and I allowed it to encroach on my life. We all know that it's bad for us. We all know it makes us smell bad, and we sure as hell know it puts a growing dent in our wallet.

So why do we not take action? Laziness, maybe? Human nature to avoid pain, maybe? Is it our busy lives in our own rat race and pressures we put on ourselves, maybe? Or is it this association with comfort tied in with an addiction to boot? It could be one or more of these things for a given individual.

But, one thing is certain, of all the different methods for quitting, be it cold turkey, be it Champex, weaning off with vaping or whatever, regardless of what your reason was to stop or try to stop, ultimately your success to quit comes down to one thing: you have to want to NOT smoke. More than you WANT to smoke at any given moment. This is where I think most of us trip up.

The first time I quit was in 1998. I was in the Army and I had a young family. I had all the right reasons to quit and I really tried to. But instead of taking breaks, I was avoiding breaks to avoid congregating with the smokers. I just worked through. My thought process was to stay busy and give the smokers a wide berth.

Initially that worked really well, but my stress levels were not in check, because I was neglecting to take breaks. It was just a matter of time before I found myself putting a cancer stick in my mouth.

The second time I quit was better than the first; however, I had not recognised fully my association of smoking with comfort. And, after a few benders with the boys, I found myself smoking again. For you non-smokers: alcohol and smoking go together like French fries and tomato sauce. Okay by themselves, but really, really, really good together.

Which brings me to my third and current 'vacation' from smoking. Having recognised the association, I've been more careful in my actions. Suffice to say it's been an evolution, not a revolution.

I can say, hand on heart, that I can be in any situation, be that of heavy drinking immersed with a group of cigarette smokers, chain-smoking in my face, and not be remotely interested in having a drag. It didn't happen overnight, but I come back to my earlier statement: you have to want to NOT smoke. More than you WANT to smoke, at any given moment.

We all have a million reasons to stop. Health, family and cost, to name a few. Here are a few ideas that worked for me, to help me quit this filthy habit:

One, make sure you keep taking breaks during the day. Manage your stress levels; this is key.

Two, tell yourself every morning your 'why' you are quitting. Set your frame of mind every day. The path you are on is a good one.

For me, I would look over at my wife asleep in bed, and the rest of my 'whys' would come to me really quickly from there.

Three, if you fall off the wagon, reset, take note of why you fell off and get back on that wagon. Make a new strategy to help yourself achieve your goal and go again. It's taken me three attempts and, no, none of them were easy. But keep reminding yourself that you want to NOT smoke, more than you WANT to smoke.

Darren Watson

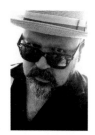

Darren Watson is a blues guitarist and singer from Wellington. In the 1980s he fronted Chicago Smoke Shop, recording two albums featuring songs he wrote, and since going solo in the 1990s he's released four highly acclaimed solo albums. He's toured with Joe Cocker, Robert Cray, Dr John, and Keb' Mo'. The blues remains his passion. From the time he was at intermediate school, he was smoking. It took a truly shocking experience for him to quit.

I was about 12 when I started smoking. You could go into a dairy and buy one or two if you wanted to in those days, so you didn't need a lot of money to get started. And that's what we did.

It got intense pretty quickly. By high school I was chuffing through half a pack a day. I bloody loved it! I really did! Right up to the day I quit I loved smoking. Even when I got sick I still loved smoking. It is a bloody insidious habit.

I'd never had asthma before, but the doctor diagnosed me with asthma. And I still chuffed away all through that. I started to have some weird effects from smoking. I was on tour with Midge Marsden, and those guys are funny, they crack you up. I would get into these laughing fits, and then not be able to breathe and I'd pass out. I did that a couple of times and still chuffed away.

It really got me once, in the studio, when I was recording. It was a song called 'Crocodile Smile', and we all had a few drinks and there was a really relaxed vibe in the studio, a late night session at Marmalade in Wellington.

We were sitting listening to a playback and somebody told this joke and I lost it. Honestly, I remember not being able to breathe, and then I just woke up on my hands and knees, dripping blood, with everyone around me saying 'My God, my God!' I'd blacked out and cut my head open on the way down. I was rushed off to hospital.

I had to have six stitches in my forehead and was on a respirator in hospital. That was the moment where I decided it was probably about time to quit! That was early 2000. It just goes to show how strong the habit is, all the other warnings I had had, and I didn't do anything about it.

I'd tried to quit three or four times before that incident. I think as much as you tell yourself you love it, it is all those other times when you are crook and it just makes it worse!

I couldn't quit. It took that massive bloody incident for me to be able to stop. I am really grateful now that it happened, because I would probably still be chuffing to this day.

I tried all the gum, I tried the patches, I tried willpower. In the end, it was this incident that convinced me. This is bad enough. That was it for me. I hope most people don't have to have an incident of that nature to wake up, but that is what it took for me.

After the incident, I just stopped. I did. For some reason, it didn't feel like a chore to stop at that point. Because I'd had such a big shock. You know when you have one of those kind of incidents, it starts to make you think about your own mortality, about how you can just be gone in a second.

I think I probably made the connection with 'if I keep this up it is going to happen again, and worse'. I tell people this all the time, it took that graphic a thing.

But hopefully, if people read about this, you don't want to be passing out when you're having a laugh or dropping where you stand. It is bloody nasty!

To this day, when I smell cigarette smoke I have that kind of double whammy of 'That smells good'. Because you have still got that addiction, and it stays with you, I think. My mother smoked all through my childhood, and you grow up around it and it's like a childhood smell.

The other thing when I smell smoke is that I get a little throb in my forehead where I hit myself! It's like my body is going 'Yeah, nah, son, don't even think about it'. It's the good angel and the bad angel.

I couldn't go back now. I think about all those times when you got a cold or the flu or something and you had to still go out and have a fag. You're bloody miserable really, but you think you're having a good time.

I don't know if my story is a typical one, probably not, but what it does say is that the stuff is poison and it is so addictive.

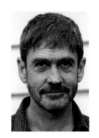

Paul Little

Paul Little is a writer, journalist, editor and publisher. He's a Herald On Sunday *columnist, and reviews New Zealand books every month in* North & South *magazine. He wrote the bestselling books,* Willie Apiata VC: The Reluctant Hero, Ray Avery: Rebel with a Cause, Paul Henry: What Was I Thinking *and* Stolen Lives: The Untold Stories of the Lawson Quins. *Before becoming a fulltime writer in 1998 he was the editor of* Metro *and the* Listener. *He produced two of his wife Wendyl Nissen's books and then formed Paul Little Books, which has published, amongst others, the series of* Grumpy Old Men *books. One of his children who urged him to stop smoking was his son Joel, the gifted musician who co-writes with, and produces, Lorde's songs.*

I would have been 16, at school, when I started smoking. It was something I had trouble not doing almost from the start, and probably accelerated quite quickly into a regular habit.

For me, smoking was always associated with reading and writing, which is mostly what I did right from university, so there was a lot of it there.

In those days, in the 1970s, there were no restrictions on where you could smoke, so you smoked in the common room. And then in my first jobs you smoked in all the offices. There was no issue about that.

Stopping? I probably tried to stop from the moment I started, or not long after. I can remember, certainly in my early 20s, trying to stop. Even before I had kids. And trying everything around. I can't think of any of the major techniques that I didn't try.

I wanted to stop because of the health issues. It didn't cost too much when I started in the mid-70s. It was 25 cents a packet or something like that. My income increased commensurate with the increased tax on cigarettes, so I was able to keep up.

I stopped when I was 50, nine years ago, and I can't remember exactly what the price of a packet of cigarettes was then, but it was nothing like as scary as it is now. I remember last year, ironically enough, visiting a friend who was dying of lung cancer. The doctors had said to her, as they do to a lot of people with lung cancer, 'Well, there's no point bothering not to smoke.' I went in to buy her a packet of fags and I didn't really know what to do. They're not on display any more. I remember being shocked at the price, whatever it was.

It is terrible, given that people have an addiction, and they just have to find that money in many cases.

The times when I tried to give up, I guess it was too easy to stop trying. My health was okay, nobody was going to leave me because of it. We were all smoking outside by that stage, so it wasn't an issue about affecting other people as much as it had been.

So I guess it was the fact that I had problems with the kids who, as far as they knew, I'd only ever been a smoker. I promised them that I would give up when I turned 50.

I was 50 and a quarter, and I still hadn't given up, and I was 50 and a half, and . . . it was all getting a bit tense.

I found out later that both they and my GP didn't actually believe that I was ever going to give up, even at that point. My GP said to me, 'I had you down as a lifelong smoker.'

I was a really committed, first thing in the morning, last thing at night cigarette smoker. I had stopped short of those people who wake up in the middle of the night and have a fag, of whom you have probably heard. I was never a chain smoker, in the sense of somebody lighting one cigarette off another.

But there were always triggers, which I understand is a big part of the nicotine addiction. I could identify what the things were that made me smoke, and they were basically everything I did. Waking up! Going to bed! All the stuff in between! Finishing a meal, reading and writing.

By then, as a journalist, you couldn't smoke at work. Although, funnily enough, when the *Listener* was in Dominion Road and I was there in 1992–94, I had an office which, for some reason, was a smoking permitted area. Robin Dudding used to come and sit in my office and smoke and read proofs. Not many other people though. That would have been the end of any smoking at work, 1994.

I certainly didn't stop on my own. One of my nearest misses was the (English writer) Allen Carr's stop smoking book. It didn't work, but it was very good. The thing that made a difference was an Allen Carr seminar that you go to, which was a separate thing. It was expensive, it was $450 or thereabouts, but if it didn't work, you got your money back. So it was very much that I had nothing to lose when I went into it, which is perhaps very revealing of my character.

I paid over my money, I went to the seminar and I've never smoked since, or even been remotely tempted. I couldn't believe it!

Why did it work for me? It was a combination of things. Most of the strategies in the book reorient your thinking about smoking, so that you don't see not smoking as missing out on something.

Which is true of a lot of addictions because you think, 'I deserve a drink. I've earned a drink. I've earned a cigarette.'

From memory, that feeling, any unpleasantness, is just the poison leaving your body, or something like that, it makes you think that.

A lot of it is common sense, but there is an element of hypnosis in it, very much suggestion. There are no trances or anything, although there was definitely a period where I wasn't really aware of what was going on around me, then I remember coming back.

I am a big advocate, mainly because for me nothing else had worked and this worked. It was nine years ago, and I've never had so much as a puff since.

I started out being quite generous towards other smokers, 'Oh, I don't mind, you go ahead and smoke.' Now I just can't stand being around smoke, as it becomes rarer and rarer, I guess.

I had been very worried, because I was working from home then and I could smoke and write all the time, and I was worried that I'd have trouble. But I just didn't.

The only problem I had was at first I did find it quite hard to concentrate, especially when reading. I went and saw a hypnotherapist, I had one session and he gave me a tape and I listened to that a few times. There has been absolutely nothing since then.

Kiwi Men's Movies

For most of us, movies are a great way to relax and escape the daily grind. Here are the favourite films of 20 Kiwi men, all of whom know what it's like to perform under some pressure in their workplace.

Kieran Read, All Blacks captain: *The Lord of the Rings* trilogy, 2001–2003, starring Elijah Wood, Sir Ian McKellen. I like the huge scale of the stories, and the epic staging of the fight scenes. The clincher is that it's shot here in New Zealand, using our amazing landscape.

John Key, former prime minister: *Avatar*, 2009, starring Sam Worthington, Zoe Saldana. My favourite because it has a really fascinating story, which is told with the most brilliant cinematography and graphic effects.

Shaun Johnson, Warrior and Kiwi, 2014 Golden Boot-winner for best league player in the world: *The Departed*, 2006, starring Leonardo DiCaprio, Jack Nicholson. A great movie with a great story, and an amazing cast, Leonardo DiCaprio, Matt Damon, Jack Nicholson and Mark Wahlberg make it a must-see.

Mike Hosking, host of NewstalkZB breakfast show, and TVNZ's *Seven Sharp*: *Love Actually*, 2003, starring Hugh Grant, Liam Neeson, Laura Linney. I like the intertwining of the stories, the clever way the characters' lives cross over, and the positive message. I cry every time.

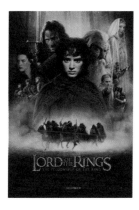 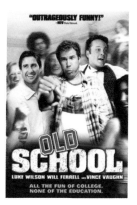 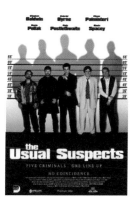

Grant Fox, All Blacks selector: *The Shawshank Redemption*, 1994, starring Tim Robbins, Morgan Freeman. I'm not much of a movie-goer, but I've probably seen this movie five or six times. I love the fact that Tim Robbins' character, by being so patient for so long, overcomes adversity and, in the process, makes sure the corrupt warden and his people are held to account for what they've done.

Simon Dallow, Television ONE newsreader: *The Usual Suspects*, 1995, starring Kevin Spacey, Gabriel Byrne. Clever, smart, complex crime thriller with great twists and turns, especially at the end. Plus a great cast with Kevin Spacey, Pete Postlethwaite and Benicio del Toro. Magnificent.

Dean Lonergan, sports promoter, former Kiwi league player: *Pulp Fiction*, 1994, starring John Travolta, Samuel L. Jackson, Uma Thurman. I think it's the greatest movie ever made. I'm a big fan of Quentin Tarantino, and with *Pulp Fiction* he made a movie that you really have to concentrate on, while at the same time entertaining the hell out of you.

Bryan Williams, All Blacks wing 1970–79: *Out of Africa*, 1985, starring Meryl Streep, Robert Redford. I'm a huge Meryl Streep fan and, as always, she was outstanding in this film. On a very personal

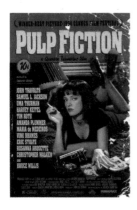 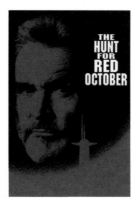 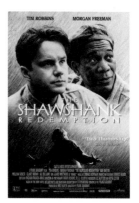

level, the amazing scenery brought back lots of memories of the first time I ever went to Africa, as a teenager in the 1970 All Blacks.

Mike McRoberts, TV3 *Newshub* newsreader: *No Country for Old Men*, 2007, starring Tommy Lee Jones, Javier Bardem. For me this film came in a nose ahead of another Coen brothers' classic, *Fargo*. Both movies have a wonderful tapestry of bloodlust, vengeance, betrayal and black humour. An adaptation of Cormac McCarthy's 2005 novel, Joel and Ethan Coen bring the book to life with suspense, wry wit and an undercurrent of hopelessness. As it turns out, West Texas is no country for anyone, let alone old men.

Nathan Astle, Black Caps batsman who hit the fastest double century in test cricket history off 153 balls, on his way to a total of 222 against England in Christchurch in 2002: *Old School*, 2003, starring Will Ferrell, Vince Vaughn, Luke Wilson. I really enjoy comedy, because the older I get the more I believe life's too short to not enjoy it. Will Ferrell's made some movies that maybe aren't so great, but I've watched *Old School* half a dozen times, and sat there laughing every time.

Greg McGee, acclaimed writer of the 2015 novel *The Antipodeans*, Richie McCaw's biography *The Open Side*, the ground-breaking 1980

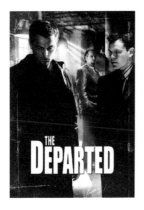
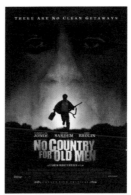
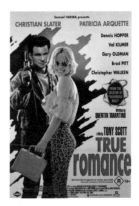

play *Foreskin's Lament*, numerous television series, and two films. And a 1972 Junior All Black: *True Romance*, 1993, starring Christian Slater, Patricia Arquette. Love story with a difference. Script by Tarantino, shot by Ridley Scott's late brother Tony, soundtrack by Hans Zimmer, cameos by the likes of Gary Oldman, Brad Pitt, Val Kilmer, Samuel L. Jackson, James Gandolfini, not to mention my favourite Christopher Walken, and Dennis Hopper, who bring alive what is one of the best drama sequences I've ever seen. Watch for the caravan and the discussion of Sicilian parentage and ask yourself why Cliff Worley (Dennis Hopper) is mentioning it.

Ian Foster, All Blacks assistant coach: *The Usual Suspects*, 1995, starring Kevin Spacey, Gabriel Byrne. It's a great yarn, and what I really like is that, as complicated as the story is, the answer is right under your nose the whole time.

Goran Paladin, presenter of *Your First Home* on ONE, Radio Sport drive show host: *Commando*, 1985, starring Arnold Schwarzenegger. Arnie plays a former commando whose young daughter, played by Alyssa Milano, is kidnapped. He has to do a lot of terrible things to get her back. It's a terrible movie really. There's one scene when Arnie is holding a guy over a cliff with one hand, and you can see in the shot the strap that's really holding the guy up. But when I was about 10 my

145

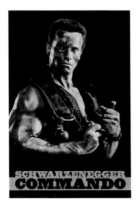 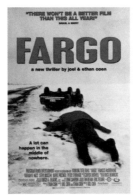 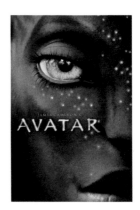

best friend Ben and I always watched it on sleepovers, so it's a movie with nothing but great memories for me.

Sir Stephen Tindall, founder of The Warehouse, philanthropist: *The Sound of Music,* 1965, starring Julie Andrews, Christopher Plummer. Call me old-fashioned but it's still *The Sound of Music.* I like it because of the heart-warming way the combination of children and music shows how a family can escape from evil. Hugely uplifting.

Wayne Shelford, undefeated All Blacks captain, 1987 World Cup winner: *Furious 7,* 2015, starring Vin Diesel, Paul Walker, Jason Statham. The scene at the end (a tribute to Paul Walker who died during the making of the film) really made an impression on me. It was a reminder that in your life the most important thing is your family.

Tony Veitch, host of 'Veitch On Sport' on NewstalkZB: *The Hunt for Red October,* 1990, starring Sean Connery, Alec Baldwin. I'm obsessed with stories about the CIA, the FBI, fascinated by the Kennedy assassinations, and have a lifetime dream to one day be in the situation room at the White House. I love spy novels, especially those written by a guy called Vince Flynn, and Thomas Clancy's Jack Ryan series. Baldwin plays Ryan in this movie, and the other lead role is played by my favourite actor, Sean Connery.

Stephen Fleming, former Black Caps captain, coach in Indian premier league and Australian Big Bash: *Old School*, 2003, starring Will Ferrell, Vince Vaughn, Luke Wilson. A very funny movie that I never get tired of. Classic one-liners and some scenes that have become cult classics. For my money, Will Ferrell is an absolute genius.

Larry Williams, drive show host on NewstalkZB: *Fargo*, 1996, starring Frances McDormand, William H. Macy. A crime thriller by the Coen brothers, with Frances McDormand as a pregnant Minnesota police chief, investigating roadside murders. Violent, quirky and darkly funny, McDormand was like a female version of Colombo, and she did it so well she won an Oscar!

Temuera Morrison, actor, whose career ranges from playing Dr Ropata in *Shortland Street* to Jake in *Once Were Warriors* to Jango Fett in *Star Wars*: *Mahana*, 2016, starring Temuera Morrison, Akuhata Keefe. I love this movie because it was such a pleasure to go to the launch in Hamilton with my aunty, who grew up in the country, and to see a movie she and other relations could relate to, not all gang stuff. It's set in the 1960s, which was a golden era for Maori, before the big move into the cities began. We won't get those years back, but it's great to see them so well portrayed. I saw it four times in quick succession and still enjoyed it.

Duncan Garner, host of MediaWorks' *The AM Show*: *Welcome to Sarajevo*, 1997, starring Woody Harrelson, Marisa Tomei. Couple of journos chasing stories in a war zone. Totally puffed up in true Hollywood style, but also based on genuine events, which interest me. And, of course, the United Nations is painted as totally hopeless and ineffective. And on that front, nothing has changed.

Depression
It's Not a Weakness

'Always remember,' says Sir John Kirwan, 'that depression is an illness, not a weakness.'

Depression respects nobody. Talent, power, fame and fortune mean nothing to it. Winston Churchill led England through World War II while struggling with what he called 'the black dog'. At the height of his career musical superstar Bruce Springsteen says he had to cope with crippling depression.

John Kirwan had the rugby world at his feet as a match-winning, try-scoring All Blacks wing. Yet, in 1991, he told his provincial coach he had to miss a game because he had the flu when, in reality, he was so depressed he could only lie in bed, shaking and crying.

John himself, by fronting television and online campaigns for mental health and producing a bestselling book, *All Blacks Don't Cry: A Story of Hope*, has helped progress the attitude of Kiwi men towards mental health. When Kirwan first mentioned his problems to footy mates when he was playing, some awkwardly suggested he 'harden up'.

There are, of course, other serious mental health issues, such as schizophrenia, where a sufferer may have the frightening experience of losing touch with reality, or bipolar disorder, involving shifts of mood, ranging from elation to bouts of extreme depression. But by far the most common mental health problems are depression and anxiety, which make up over 90% of mental illnesses in New Zealand. If you're troubled by depression, you're not alone. One in eight Kiwi men will

148

suffer from it at some stage of their lives.

What are the signs that how you feel is more than a 'bad day at the office', but actual clinical depression?

Keep in mind that depression is never as clear cut as a broken bone that can be x-rayed, or blood pressure that can be physically measured. All depressions are slightly different. But psychotherapist Kyle MacDonald says there are things to look out for.

'Probably the number-one big red flag for men would be anger. A lot of people don't know that often anger is a symptom of depression for guys.

'In a broader sense, I would say if you find yourself doing, or saying things, that you regret or don't feel good about. That could be yelling at your wife, yelling at your kids. It could be missing work deadlines. It could be just missing commitments, missing catching up with mates, or important appointments. If you feel your behaviour starting to slip.

'So it's one thing to have a bad day, but when we get to that point where we just feel tired all the time, or we're disengaging or withdrawing. If you're struggling to get any enjoyment out of things then I think that's often a really good red flag that something is going on.'

There's a clinical name for that state, anhedonia, an absence of pleasure.

'When we start to just feel like life is a bit flat. We can't really get excited about anything. We feel burnt out and tired. Like the batteries are just running a bit flat.'

It could be that the trouble will be resolved without medical intervention.

'You may solve the problem, by getting a new job, or figuring out what's going wrong in your relationship, or whatever the stress in your life might be, and it passes. The problem is when people get stuck in that place, and when you get stuck in that place, then you actually end up being less able to make the changes you need to make.'

Where should you look for help?

There are a number of good online sites, with practical advice. They're listed at the end of the chapter.

If you'd rather not self-diagnose, or feel you need face-to-face assistance, Kyle MacDonald says your doctor (GP) is always a good first stop.

'The key thing with GPs is that they're pretty busy, so I often advise people if they're going to talk about something a bit complicated like, "I think I'm depressed" or "I'm drinking too much" or "I keep yelling at my wife and I don't want to", book a double appointment that gives you half an hour.'

What's likely to happen if your GP believes you need help for depression?

Like depression itself, that may vary. You may be immediately prescribed antidepressant drugs by your GP. Or you may be referred to a specialist. Or there may be a prescription and a referral.

It'd be a good time now to explain in broad terms the difference between the mental health specialists, the people who may be your next stop after seeing your GP.

A psychiatrist is likely to be dealing with the more extreme forms of mental illness, such as schizophrenia. He or she will have first spent five years obtaining a medical degree, then have worked for two years as a supervised junior doctor in a hospital, and finally spent five years of specialised training to qualify as a psychiatrist. Because of his or her medical qualifications, a psychiatrist can prescribe drugs.

A psychologist will have a Masters, or higher, university degree in psychology, and have had at least 1500 hours supervised work, approved and evaluated by the New Zealand Psychologists Board. He or she cannot prescribe drugs, but can make recommendations to your GP.

A psychotherapist will have a diploma or Masters degree in psychotherapy, and will have met qualifications and work experience criteria for registration with the Psychotherapists Board of Aotearoa New Zealand. Like a psychologist, he or she cannot prescribe drugs, but can make recommendations to your GP.

There's no clear direction in New Zealand on what course of action is best for mild to moderate depression, although the American Psychiatric Association and the British National Institute for Health and Care Excellence both recommend the first line of treatment should be 'talk therapy' rather than medication.

'There's a big variation in terms of how well connected GPs are with referral networks when it comes to talk therapy,' says Kyle MacDonald. 'It's not necessarily on top of their minds a lot of the time.'

If you decide you want to visit a psychotherapist, the websites at the end of this chapter are a good place to seek them out.

'It's entirely possible to look up a psychotherapist and make an appointment. You don't need a referral, you don't have to go through your GP. You can just book an appointment and go and have a chat with someone.'

What's most likely to happen if you go to a psychotherapist, or a clinical psychologist? One of the first things will be to discover what's triggering your depression or anxiety.

'The balanced view these days is that there are always multiple factors that contribute,' says Kyle. 'There is some evidence that some people are born with a propensity for having mood disturbances, in the same way there's evidence that some people have a propensity for anxiety.

'But we know that all sorts of things can happen in childhood that can set people up for depression. Things such as emotional neglect, emotionally distant parents, physical abuse, sexual abuse, big disruptions such as messy divorces. Bullying is another big one.

'The best way to think about it is that it's always a balance of factors, so some people might have quite a heavy genetic component, particularly when you get the severe mood disorders like bipolar. Some people might have quite a heavy environmental component, so they may have no one in their family who's ever had depression, but they've had an absolutely awful childhood.

'One of the things that I always struggle with a bit is the way that depression is talked about in the media it sometimes never quite gets across the complexity.

'If someone has had depression, when you sit down and you talk to them and they tell you about their life, and what's happened to them, it always makes sense [that they suffered depression].'

It's also possible, if you're seeing a psychologist or psychotherapist, they'll give you a recommendation for medication to take to your GP to be prescribed.

'The clinical literature is pretty clear,' says Kyle. 'It says that, in broad brush terms, with severe depression the combination of medication and therapy is one plus one equals three. So they're more effective together than either are on their own.

'When you dig into it a bit further, what it seems to say is that for mild to moderate depression, talk therapy on its own is more effective than medication. For severe depression, they're more effective together. So the best clinical advice is, if it's mild to moderate, try talk therapy first, and if that doesn't work add medication and/or see a different therapist.

'Because that's the other really important thing for people who are new to therapy, the most important factor with a therapist is just feeling like it's the right person to talk to. We call it the "therapeutic alliance". All the studies about effectiveness say really clearly that it doesn't matter what the training background is, it doesn't matter what modality or theory your therapist has, if it's a good match and a good fit and they're properly trained in something, then the therapy will be effective.'

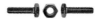

The website of the Mental Health Foundation is a wonderful resource, covering all aspects of mental health: mentalhealth.org.nz

If you are in an emergency situation, where you believe you, or someone else, is at risk, the foundation recommends the following:

Ring 111 in an emergency.

Go to the emergency department of your nearest hospital.

Phone your district health board crisis team. You can call Healthline on 0800 611 116.

If you need to speak to someone call:

Lifeline 0800 543 354 or 09 522 2999

Suicide Prevention Hotline 0508 828 865 (0508 TAUTOKO)

Youthline 0800 376 633

Samaritans 0800 726 666

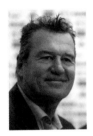

Sir John Kirwan

Sir John Kirwan astonished many New Zealanders when he revealed, in his 1992 biography Running On Instinct, *that he had suffered from depression during much of his All Blacks career. Since then he has become the much-respected face of men's mental health in New Zealand, heading highly successful campaigns to help men struggling with depression or mental illness.*

The spectrum of mental illness is wide. You can be mildly depressed at some time in your life. It might last a little while, and you don't really need any medication, or anything like that.

Then there is what happened to me. You're a normal person going along and then, through a series of events, and they could be varied, you fall into what is called a medical depression.

Anxiety and medical depression can be caused by all sorts of different factors. What I try to tell people is that depression is an illness, not a weakness.

The only trouble is that with our brain, when we start having some down times or some anxiety, a lot of people don't reach out and get help and understand the illness. It is like any other illness, the quicker you get it seen to, the more you can understand it, and the better off you will be. For example, if I had got help when I first started getting anxiety attacks when I was 18 or 19 and understood it, then quite possibly I might not have fallen into a medical depression.

Mine was a depression triggered by anxiety. If initially I had got on top of the anxiety I might not have fallen into depression. They are two separate illnesses, so people can go along in their life and have anxiety, without becoming depressed, although they are pretty closely linked. A lot of the time people who have anxiety do get depressed.

I eventually did reach out to get help. I went to this woman, whose name was Louise Armstrong, a fantastic person. I'd been to a couple of people earlier and they were just not my type of people. I went and sat down with Louise and she said to me, 'JK, if you had a tight hamstring what would you do?' I said, 'Well, I'd stop and stretch it.' She said, 'If you got up and kept running and it got really, really tight, what would you do?' I said, 'I'd ice it and go and see the physio.' She said, 'Your brain is no different.'

That really simplified it for me and I thought that is good, I've got a hamstring as a brain! I've got a hamstring in the brain and I need to ice it, and what does that ice look like?

The mistake that we often make is that we don't reach out early enough. I should have reached out straight away. But I sort of hid it for a long time instead of reaching out and getting help.

Part of the reason why I did the campaign is because if you reach out and get help early, it is like any other illness. Once I realised I had a hamstring in the head, that sort of made sense to a young rugby player. When you explain that to people, they start getting it. Okay, it is an illness, I can reach out and get some help. How do I deal with this? I try to simplify it for people.

I was pretty bad by the time I got to Louise Armstrong. I was really unwell. I had to medicate, which I didn't like. But that was stupid too, because we go to the doctor if we've got the flu, we jam whatever they give us down our throats.

My dad was really good. I was standing next to him at the bench one day. I said, 'Dad I hate taking this bloody thing for the head.' He turned to me and said, 'Do you want me to die do you?' I said, 'No.' And he said, 'Well, I've got to take 22 of these little buggers and if I don't I'll be dead tomorrow.' He was talking about his heart pills. That got me over myself a wee bit.

Then I thought I needed to get some balance back into my life, which I did. I started working on the illness which involved some techniques for which the technical phrase is 'cognitive behaviour therapy'. I just called it 'rewiring the brain'.

So I worked on rewiring the brain and looked for stuff that would keep me well every day, and I sort of started again, which is a really cool thing to do when you see the end results.

People often ask me if I'm worried about getting depressed again, and the answer is no, because I took all the fear out of it, all the fear out of the anxiety, and all the fear out of the depression. What I did learn was to look after myself. So I look after myself every day. What does that mean? That means I know that every day I've got to read, or work out in the gym, or do whatever works for me. When I say to people 'wellness is every day' I really mean it. You have got to be able to know what to do every day to keep yourself well.

ONE FROM DAD

Paul Ego is one of the stars of TV3's 7 Days, *a successful radio breakfast show host and a popular stand-up comedian. You'll have also heard him doing the voice of Stickman on the PAK'nSAVE TV commercials. Paul says he's not really a joke teller, but says he loves this one his dad told him recently.*

A guy was out hunting and he tripped, firing his shotgun into his groin. His friends got him to hospital and, when he woke, a male doctor and a woman were standing over his bed.

'What happened?' he asked.

The doctor told him he'd shot himself in the groin with buckshot, but said that they'd managed to remove all the buckshot and save his penis.

Relieved, the hunter looked at the woman and said, 'Who's this?'

The doctor said, 'Well, we DID manage to remove all the pellets from your penis but there will be an adjustment period. This lady is going to help you with that.'

'Is she a psychologist or something?' said the hunter.

'No,' said the doctor. 'She plays the flute for the Philharmonia. She's gonna show you where to put your fingers so you don't piss in your eye.'

Great Food
That Doesn't Taste Like Crap

Fitness expert Lee-Anne Wann lives and breathes good health. You may have seen her on TVNZ's Kiwi Living *show, heard her on the radio or read one of her books,* Downsize You *or* No-Fuss Fitness. *In 2013 she was appointed the Vodafone Warriors' nutritionist. A hugely successful series in the* New Zealand Herald, *where she helped four Kiwi men to make big changes to their lives and wellbeing, led to her appointment as an Ambassador for the New Zealand Men's Health Trust. Down to earth, with a great sense of humour, Lee-Anne is a huge advocate for men's health.*

Eating well and being healthy isn't complicated. In fact, it's really just a case of going back to the basics. As we have evolved we look for better things, new solutions, an innovative approach, but we may be missing out on the basics.

As men today, you put a lot of pressure on yourselves. There is still that traditional approach where you are out there having to support the family and facing complex problems at work.

Through nutrition, let's look at ways to support that. Let's keep things simple. And let's be consistent. You are the sum of what you do consistently, not on occasion.

Why does breakfast matter?

Start with the fundamentals, those things we underestimate, something as simple as getting up in the morning and eating breakfast.

How many men don't do that? We're all told, eat breakfast. But, as a man, always looking for a reason and for a solution, you'll probably ask: 'Why?'

Because if you want to improve your focus, your clarity and your concentration, then choosing not only to eat breakfast, but to eat a certain type of food, will influence and have an impact on your performance. We all want to be that 2%, 5% or 10% better than our competition.

Eating the right breakfast not only helps with your performance during the day, but also with your long-term health. It's all about bang for your buck. If you choose to take a small portion of time and allocate it to your health, your wellbeing, and your performance, you want to choose the period of time that will have the most impact. In my opinion, that's the morning.

If you take 10 minutes to eat a breakfast higher in protein, that will affect the neurotransmitters or chemical messengers in your brain that in turn affect focus, drive and concentration. It also helps control your appetite and your energy levels throughout the day. It helps with detoxification. It helps you combat life.

If you start your day with sugary cereals or if you choose something highly processed that your body can't get what it needs out of, then you are not going to function as well as you could. Ultimately that will cause damage to your hormone, health and stress levels, which can be one of the biggest problems in maintaining good health.

You need to eat actual food, not food out of packets. We need to eat the food that nature intended us to eat. It is not dieting; it is not counting calories; it is not saying eat loads of this or that. It is just actual food. Real food.

What makes a great breakfast?

We all need a variety of foods. If you want to make breakfast easy, it could be something like leftover dinner. If you have a steak that is left over, have a couple of eggs with it. Or if you had some chicken left over, have it with some broccoli. I believe leftover dinner is a man's best breakfast. It's easy, quick and requires no great planning or thought. Let's be honest, nobody wants to cook loads of things in the morning.

The other option is having eggs. Eggs are brilliant. People say, 'I get a bit bored with eggs.' Okay, try them different ways. Poached eggs are very different from scrambled eggs, which are different from an omelette, which is different to a boiled egg. If you like tomatoes have some with eggs.

Eggs are a good source of branched-chain amino acids. They are a particularly healthy component for your liver. Most of all, they're just real food.

If occasionally you run out of time or run out of eggs, stop at a café, and ask them for bacon and eggs. Bacon is not perfect by any means, but pick your battles. Is that better, on occasion, and closer to the natural source, than some coloured sugary loops out of a box?

Even if you're not a breakfast eater, have a couple of Brazil nuts in the morning. Our soil is selenium deficient and Brazil nuts are a good source of selenium, which acts an as antioxidant and also helps regulate blood pressure.

As a man, how do you make the decisions about, and what are the results of, putting certain fuels into your body? It's like putting a premium fuel into your motor vehicle. When you go to the service station you don't put diesel in a petrol car. Because it is not going to run. You don't put in low-grade petrol unless you have to. Why? Because your car runs better on high octane. This is the same principle for you in the morning.

You want to run well for that entire day? Then you choose the best food you have on hand and then, if you have a choice, you choose the best protein, because that affects not only those chemical messengers of focus and drive but also protein synthesis, muscle regeneration and growth.

If you change nothing else in your day, but decide to eat a good-quality, protein-rich breakfast, in my book that is 50% of the battle done.

What's the miracle on tap in your home?

When you wake up in the morning you've gone for a long period of sleeping without food on board.

Here's a big tip, an almost magical health provider that in New Zealand is easily available, because it's literally on tap. Water. It's cheap, it's easy, and in this country (with the odd sad exception like the contamination problems in Havelock North) it's mostly clean and safe.

When you sleep you become dehydrated and levels of cortisol, the stress hormone, are elevated. Cortisol is the hormone that wakes you up in the morning. We want to bring those levels down, and they will come down when you're hydrated.

Water is the most underrated thing.

As men get older with joint issues, an aching back, not enough energy to get out of bed, a headache, feeling really average, all these things guys push to one side because they need to carry on, water will help with them all.

Think about the last time you had a hangover. What helped? What did your body crave? Water.

If you only have 10 minutes to spare in the morning, drink some water. It helps with nearly every bodily function. If all you do in the morning when you get up is eat breakfast and drink some water, I know that's not very exciting. In fact, it is very unexciting. It certainly doesn't seem to be a miracle pill, does it? But it is. In some ways, I wouldn't even categorise water as a drink; it is a life requirement, like breathing.

Here's another really simple, but hugely effective, tip. Try adding some chia seeds to your water. If you've never heard of them, they look like little black poppy seeds. You get them from the bulk bins

160

in the supermarket, and they're cheap. They are an ancient Indian running food from the Americas. The Aztec people supposedly used to use them to help with endurance and energy. They would just have these grains and eat them while they went for a three-day run.

The reason I like them is because they are hydrophilic; they absorb up to eight to nine times their weight in fluid.

If you can't drink as much as you should, or if hydration is something you'd like to focus on, adding chia seeds to your water or to your food will improve your hydration levels. I use them for the Warriors when we fly, because jetlag is mostly caused by dehydration.

Looking at bang for your buck, do you care if you put a tablespoon of chia seeds into your water throughout the day? Maybe not. But the impact on the body is profound. It is the sum of all these little things that will help you.

How do you meet your water goal?

I'm picking you'll want, as men often do, some facts and figures . . .

A really good idea is to have a water goal. What should it be? You'll have heard a lot of numbers thrown around. The magic goal of eight eight-ounce glasses a day has been around for years. That's almost two litres a day. The American Institute of Medicine recommends even more, about three litres a day for men. Another aim that's been suggested is about 40ml per kilo. So, if you're 100kg, that's four litres a day, which is a huge amount.

I'm certainly not disrespecting those messages. But I'd suggest aiming for 1.5 litres a day, and, here's the key, being consistent with it.

Don't be intimidated by the idea of four litres a day. To be honest, if you drink that much you'll be peeing all the time. Back off a little bit, and do the 1.5 litres every day.

What will help you make sure you drink that much water

consistently? Let's think first about what will work for you and set some goals.

The first thing 99% of people do in the morning is drink some water. Let's make that first drink 500ml (2 cups). Then, after breakfast and a shower, drink another 500ml before you leave the house. There's a litre done.

If you're office based, get a bottle of water and put it on your desk. You'll know just by looking at it whether you're drinking enough. Or you might set an alarm on your phone to remind you to take a drink.

What if you get bored with water?

During the day, you might think about drinking sparkling water, which is very different to plain water. My father found this out. He was bored with water and he doesn't really drink coffee. He might have tea now and again.

I said, 'Dad why don't you try sparkling water?' He said, 'It's expensive. I'm not having that; it's just stupid.'

Then he tried it. Oh my goodness. He started hunting down this particular size of sparkling water, in the small bottles, because it stays sparkling and he thinks it is amazing. He said to me, 'Who would have thought that it would be so refreshing and just different on the palate.' In the end I bought him a SodaStream so he could make his own, obviously without the syrups.

Sparkling water, as long as it doesn't have sugar added, is as good as drinking pure, plain water.

Do be careful with bottled sparkling water, to make sure it has not got added flavours. The marketers are very clever. They take a good clean product and then slightly adjust it. They will put in something that is a little bit addictive. They look for the bliss point in foods that causes you to crave more.

You don't find a sign over the broccoli in the supermarket that says 'Buy one and go into the draw to win $10,000.' You just don't. We don't need enticing, because we know these things are good for us.

What's the issue with soft drinks?

The trouble with fizzy drinks is that they contain such large quantities of sugar. I'd suggest making gradual changes. Maybe swap one fizzy drink with plain water, and go from there.

Iced tea in bottles is presented as something that is healthy, but it often has large quantities of sugar in it.

Green tea that you make yourself, without sugar, is very good for you. It can help reduce blood pressure. It helps reduce cortisol, the stress hormone. It helps with burning fat and it also helps with detoxification.

There are so many compelling reasons to drink green tea that you might decide, even if you don't love it, that you'll have a cup at morning tea for the health benefits alone.

How can I check that a drink is healthy?

If you're unsure about any form of drink, the ingredients labels are quite challenging to read. Here's a simple but very good rule. Just turn it over and look at the sugar per serve listing. If it's three grams or less, that's good. Anything over five grams per serve and you're getting up there. So, if it's seven grams, you make the call. If it's 25 grams, please think twice — do you really want that much sugar in your body?

As far as coffee is concerned, I'm not against it. Black coffee helps with concentration. If you do drink coffee and you regularly drink, say, a mochaccino with chocolate syrup, I would try to reduce the amount of sugar you are consuming with your coffee.

What about fruit juices?

You're better off eating an orange than drinking orange juice. Orange juice is full of sugar, a very condensed source of fructose, which is not ideal.

If you eat an apple instead of drinking apple juice you get the fibre and nutrients without an overload of sugar as you get with juice.

Even carrot juice is worth thinking twice about. It takes about 10 carrots to make a glass of juice. Would you eat 10 carrots? The food itself is not bad, it's what we've done to it.

What's best to keep muscles working?

As we age, our muscles degenerate. We lose muscle mass from the age of 20 or so. We want to protect our muscle mass and we can help do that by how we eat. When we don't get nutrients, when we don't get good food, our body taps into our own muscle stores, so we want to avoid that.

As we get older the muscles are our shock absorbers, they determine our metabolic rate and, in doing so, protect your health. You want to protect your lean mass, your muscle mass.

You want to have again, the least processed food possible.

If you have only breads and cereals in the morning, you get sugar and carbohydrates. These cause the body to produce serotonin and dopamine, which will make you sleepy and tired, and that is not what you want in the morning or during the day.

The most simple advice is actually the most profound: if your food doesn't have an ingredients list, it's probably good for you.

If it has an ingredients label it's been manufactured and processed. These are products masquerading as foods. They are okay on occasion, but as your stock standard fuel for great health, vitality, energy, performance, the most nutrient-dense food is your best choice. And the most nutrient dense is typically the most natural. So eat a potato instead of a hash brown. What's more natural? It came out of the ground.

A lot of these products are advertised in mainstream media and they're in the supermarkets, so they must be okay, right? It is not until somebody asks you to question those products that you start to think, 'These are products that are like food, but they're still products.' If they're not products, how do they last on the shelf for so long? Natural is always going to be best.

Should I be afraid of fats?

In moderation, nothing is terrible for you. But if you are going to do something regularly you want it in a way that the body can best use it. Don't be afraid of including good, natural fats in your diet: eggs, nuts, avocado. I think that we have become quite fearful of fats, and it's not good for us.

I am an advocate of natural butter, which is particularly good for men's health.

That doesn't mean that you should go overboard with it, and it doesn't mean that you should fry all your food in it.

Your brain is 60% saturated fat. If you want your brain to function properly, you need to eat good natural fats. The components in natural butter are very good. Butter is rich in the most easily absorbable form of vitamin A, necessary for prostate and adrenal health, contains arachidonic acid (AA), which plays a role in brain function, and is a vital component of cell membranes, as well as being a host to many other healthy nutrients.

By comparison margarine and artificial spreads are loaded with additives. So what is your best natural source of fats? Butter. All they do is churn it.

I'm talking about the butter that comes wrapped in paper. I was talking to the Warriors about putting butter on their vegetables to help with appetite. One of the boys said, 'Do you mean the cooking butter that is wrapped in paper?' I thought, 'That shows my age!' But this is what is happening: we have forgotten to stay with the basics.

How do you deal with a sweet tooth?

You pick your battles. Look at what you enjoy, and go for the most minimally processed. Avoid highly processed sweets. And be warned, if the label says something like '99% fat free', that often means it's high in sugar.

If I was choosing ice-cream it would be full fat. Some people have their own ice-cream makers, and they get full fat milk and put in fruit. That's great but not something to have too often.

What is very interesting is that if you start your day well with a protein-rich breakfast that sweet craving is less likely to occur. If you put a little bit of butter on your vegetables at dinner you probably won't have that craving for something sweet after dinner. If you have beautiful cooked salmon with the skin on, then you won't want large servings of sweet food.

It is not a question of avoiding any macronutrient, it is about optimising their use. I think that things like a little bit of dark chocolate, a bit of ice-cream, good natural stuff, is fine. The key words are 'a little bit'. Just have what you enjoy.

If you find you're really craving sweets at night, use it as a sign that something is off.

Is it because you didn't drink any water during the day? Is it because you started your day with a sugary cereal? Is it because you were in meetings all day and you skipped meals and now your body wants glucose? Are you highly stressed and agitated? What can you change to get things back on course?

What's best for an evening meal?

People are a bit fearful of carbohydrates. They think, 'Potato and kumara are bad.' But adding them to your dinner, in reasonable amounts, is great. They release serotonin and dopamine, and they both help you sleep, and they make you feel better.

If you have them with a little bit of butter, or the little bit of fat that comes from your meat, they will help you feel full, satisfied and relaxed.

You're reloading your body with fuel stores for the next day. It's a little like going to a petrol station and fuelling up. You're filling the tank at night ready for tomorrow. You don't want to fuel the tank with fuel in the morning, you want to have it done the night before and in the morning you're just doing an oil check, and getting the neurotransmitters driving.

Remember always that it's what you do consistently that matters. And without fail, if you do the little things, whether it's having a good breakfast, drinking more water, avoiding fake foods that are heavily processed, or cutting down on sugar, they will add up to a terrifically large sum.

Diabetes
Handling the Enemy Within

Diabetes is a silent assassin, an internal Ninja that might be with you from birth, or may emerge stealthily at any stage during your lifetime.

Thankfully, if you don't present an easy target, it'll never get a chance to attack, and you'll avoid it for the whole of your life. At worst, with treatment, you'll be able to stop it being lethal, and live a full, active life.

So how do you elude the diabetes assassin?

Let's have a look first at what diabetes actually is. The one to keep at bay as an adult is Type 2 diabetes, which is the kind that affects 90% of people with diabetes. To keep it simple, we'll just call it T2 from now on. (We'll look at Type 1 diabetes later.)

It all starts with your pancreas, a long, flattened gland located deep in the belly, somewhere between your stomach and your spine. The other part of the pancreas curves around your duodenum (the first part of the small intestine). To get a very good idea of where it is, and how big it is, make an 'O for Awesome' sign with your right hand. First finger and thumb circled, the other three fingers straight. Put your hand in the middle of your belly just below your lower ribs, with your straight fingers pointed to the left. Your hand is now mirroring the right shape and position of your pancreas inside your body.

So it's hidden away, but what the pancreas does is the key to avoiding T2. The pancreas produces a hormone called insulin, which allows your body to use glucose for energy, and even to store it for future use. Glucose is a form of sugar, and when everything's working properly, your body uses it in the form of blood sugar for everything from something as basic as keeping you warm, to unleashing energy. When Nick Willis kicks at the end of a 1500 metres race, healthy levels of blood sugar are providing the fuel for him.

Like so many parts of your body, a healthy pancreas is a brilliant machine. As blood sugar levels rise, as they do after eating, the pancreas secretes more insulin to keep those levels in a normal range.

Where things go haywire is if the pancreas doesn't produce enough insulin, or the cells in the body don't recognise the insulin that is present. The end result is the same: high levels of glucose in your blood.

Untreated diabetes isn't pleasant. You pick up skin infections easily, and they, as well as cuts, take a long time to heal. You may have poor eyesight, or blurred vision. Diabetes can also cause leaking fluids in your eye that affect vision. Perhaps worst of all, it can damage the kidneys and nerves in the feet and heart, sometimes with fatal consequences.

T2 lurks in the shadows and, to the untrained eye, is very hard to spot. 'It's a sneaky disorder because it creeps up on people,' says Rick Cutfield, a clinical director of endocrinology and diabetes at the Waitemata District Health Board, a life member of Diabetes New Zealand, a former president and life member of the New Zealand Society for the Study of Diabetes, and the Patron of Diabetes New Zealand (Auckland branch).

'You sometimes get symptoms like loss of energy, but who doesn't get tired at 55? Peeing in the night, but who doesn't have a pee at 65 in the middle of the night? And thirst, and so forth.

'Sometimes you have more dramatic symptoms with blurred vision and skin infections, but quite a lot of people have very subtle symptoms, that you and I would pass off as a bit of a stressful week, or a stressful month, or things not adding up at home, and so you just put it down to that.

'So it can be a very subtle slow increase in problems, which I think is why Diabetes New Zealand in most of our guidelines suggest that we can't trust ourselves with our own diagnosis of the symptoms.

'It's fine if you can recognise them, but the best thing is that regular bloke's check. Where you go at a certain age, which will maybe start at 40, and you have your check which includes your cardiovascular check.

'While it's true diabetes is glucose-centric, it's not all about sugar. It's a blood pressure, cholesterol, blood sugar conglomerate of things, so you need to check them all.

'Part of a general men's health check would include cholesterol levels, your blood pressure, and then we'll chuck in the diabetes check as well.

'And that's often now how it's being picked up, where in the old days people would just wait until they were half crook. You'd find then that 10% of people, or even up to 20% of people, by the time they got to their doctor, were already having significant complications. They'd either have coronary disease, or some patchy changes in their eyes.'

You're not alone if you find you have T2. One in 20 men in New Zealand will have it during their lifetime.

T2 is not only sneaky, but it's also racist. If you're of European descent you're most likely to get it after you turn 40. If you're of Maori, Asian, Middle Eastern or Pasifika descent, you enter the T2 danger zone earlier, at 30. Sadly those ages are heading down, with some teenagers now being diagnosed with T2.

It's worth checking your family history too. If there is a close relative who has T2 there will be a greater chance of you getting it.

What can you do to stop T2 from even arriving?

The fitter you are the better. And, along with regular exercise, not eating fattening foods is a big help too. We joke about spare tyres or love handles, but the less stomach that rolls over your belt, the less chance of your pancreas malfunctioning, and of getting T2. High blood pressure often goes along with T2, and that's often associated with weight.

As with every disease we've discussed in this book, if you do have T2 the earlier it's diagnosed the better. The longer you leave it, says Rick Cutfield, the more chances your beta cells, the insulin-producing cells, are going to get permanently wrecked.

'It does appear that the higher the sugars, the longer they are at a higher level, the more toxic they are to the remaining beta cells. It's about early and quite aggressive treatment.'

If it's caught at an early stage, one of the first issues in managing it is likely to be losing some weight. Don't panic at the thought of living for the last 30 or more years of your life on lettuce and tofu salad.

Rick has encouraging news. 'Let's say that you're 100kg. You played a bit of footy in your day, then gave it up and put on some weight. A dietitian may come up and say, "Your ideal body weight is 72kg." Then you think, "I'll never be able to lose 28kg."

'But the worst thing to do is to say you have to lose something like 30kg. You don't. And no matter how you tried, you probably wouldn't be able to anyway.

'You can still be a fat bloke at the end of it but if you've lost 5 or 10kg, which may be 5 to 10% of your weight, then it's possible your diabetes can be kept in remission.

'It's not cured, because it could come back, but if you use the word "remission" then, in other words, you're in control. You've got it. You've sort of half beaten it, and then you've just got to keep an eye on it.

'The key thing is to stick with a food plan that's not too challenging for you, because if you go on an extreme diet, you'll only do it for three months and then you'll go back to your old ways. The bottom line is to reduce calories slowly and to get a bit of advice. There's a lot of website advice, but mostly people know what to eat.

They know what they're doing wrong. It's usually overeating and the answer is just cutting down meal size, and getting rid of the simple sugars, the soft drinks and the sweets.

'It's quite easy to lose the first three or four kilos. It's a bit harder to lose the next three or four, but that may be all you need. It's a simple message, and it's a realistic message: Lose a bit of weight and get out and do some exercise.

'I've seen rugby and league players who lose two or three or four kilos and what you find is that they feel better immediately. Three months later their sugars have come down a bit, they're eating a bit better and you say, "How do you actually feel?" and they say, "I don't think I've felt better for ages."

'Sometimes you say to an ex-sportsman, "Are you doing any sport?" and he'll reply, "Nah, I've got a buggered knee from rugby" or something like that. I'll say, "Well, there's plenty of other things to do." You don't have to go to the gym. There are lots of other things to do with a bit of equipment or walking.

'The simple message is to do some exercise, something that you find enjoyable, and can do with your mates or your family, and to have a realistic weight loss plan.'

What if weight loss and exercise aren't enough?

'There's a fair percentage of people who will need tablets, and the first tablet that's used quite frequently in general practice, and works quite well, is Metformin.

'Now people may think, "Bloody tablets. I don't want to take a tablet. I'm much better than this." What I do is tell them, a little sneakily, that it's based on a French lilac. And that's true, it really does come from a plant. So it's sort of organic, and the best thing is, it works.

'If you take this tablet twice a day, one in the morning, then one at night with food, it will help control T2, and there's good evidence that it does that.

'It's a good drug. You may later have to go onto a second drug, or even a third oral tablet, and some people will go on and need insulin.'

Say insulin, and many of us think needles. Think needles and some strong men feel queasy. Rick swears nobody should be afraid of insulin. Yes, it has to be taken by way of an injection. 'That's because it gets destroyed in the stomach if you give it in tablet form. They are trying to create an insulin tablet but at the moment there isn't another way of doing it.

'But you really don't need to be afraid. It's given just under the skin. The needles are so tiny. They're 4mm long (that's about one-third the length of an eyelash) and are so thin that you can barely see them. They are basically painless. The only thing is that psychologically you have to bear putting it in, but it doesn't hurt.

'One of the things I talk to doctors and patients about is that you cannot have diabetes if you have enough insulin in your body. If you've got enough you're fine.'

Reasonably enough some men ask why they have T2, and need insulin, while their tubby mate, who might be 140kg, strolls through life never affected by diabetes.

'There may be something about your own pancreas,' says Rick. 'Your personal Bank of Insulin in your pancreas doesn't have enough deposit in it, so you've got a shortage. Or you may have been born with some sort of problem with the release of that insulin. That's why some fat people can get away with it, because they've got a very nice release mechanism.

'The gene or the abnormality that causes the problem is about either the amount of insulin that comes out of your pancreas not being enough, or the insulin not working properly, what's called "insulin resistance".'

Please don't feel that if you've drawn the unlucky pancreas function card then your weight doesn't matter. If you've inherited from your mum or dad a pancreas that isn't functioning properly, then the bigger your belly, the worse it'll function.

Fat around your belly doesn't just make Speedos a no-go zone for you, but what it does inside your body is creepy.

'If it just stayed there, it'd be okay but it's not inert,' says Rick. 'It's actually an active organ, and it produces fatty acids, which are sort of like a slime, if you like, that infiltrates other organs.

'If we overeat, and we're over-nourished, and we don't need it, the body decides to store it somewhere else. This fat then goes into the liver, and then it goes around the pancreas, and around the heart, just spreads around. So when you do scans you find fat on all these organs, and when you lose weight it disappears.

'It seems that if you're fat around your middle, you're much more predisposed to diabetes.'

If you are diagnosed with T2, Diabetes New Zealand has some very practical words of advice.

Take time out so you can have space within which to make the emotional and practical adjustments you need.

Talk to others. Share your thoughts and feelings with your friends and family. Spend time with those who can support you and understand your feelings. Talk to other people with diabetes. Their insights will help you and it's important for you to know that you are not alone. You'd be surprised how many people have it. (As of December 2015, there were 129,832 men diagnosed with diabetes in New Zealand.)

Take time to learn the skills you need to manage your diabetes. But remember you can't learn it all at once. Don't be too hard on yourself. Take it one step at a time.

See a dietitian to get the most up-to-date information and support for your food choices.

Attend local diabetes groups or classes or visit a diabetes nurse educator.

Make contact with your local diabetes organisation to see if they run support groups or have other resources. If you find living with diabetes especially hard have some counselling.

When you do make changes to your lifestyle, don't try doing it all at once. One manageable step at a time is best. And don't forget to give yourself a pat on the back when you achieve each step.

Now let's look at Type 1, a much rarer type of diabetes. How rare? Put 200 Kiwi men in a room, and about nine will have T2 diabetes. One will have T1 diabetes.

'Type 1 is nobody's fault,' says Rick. 'It's a genetic disorder which you are either lucky enough to miss, or unlucky enough to get. It can skip generations.

'People used to call it youth diabetes, or similar things, because they thought that only children and teenagers got it. But it turns out that the prevalence of Type 1 diabetes is identical in every decade. You can get it at any age.'

It is different from T2 diabetes in that insulin is needed to treat T1 from the beginning. Tablets don't work, and T1 needs more detailed management in terms of juggling insulin, food and exercise.

The harsh reality is that people with diabetes don't live quite as long as people without it. But the life expectancy of someone with diabetes is improving dramatically all the time, as is how people cope with diabetes.

'Diabetes doesn't respect rank or fame,' says Rick Cutfield. 'There are leaders of industry, and former great sports stars, people who are household names, who use insulin every day, and are leading very normal lives, and coping very well.

'The fact is that today people can live a good, full and healthy life with diabetes.'

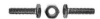

Diabetes New Zealand is a charitable organisation that's been at work for more than 50 years. Their extensive website is at: diabetes.org.nz.

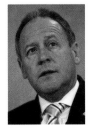

Sir Ralph Norris

Sir Ralph Norris is one of New Zealand's most successful and respected businessmen. But Type 2 diabetes, he believed, was leaving him so exhausted that when he retired from his position as chief executive of the ASB Bank he never dreamed that within months he would be taking over as CEO and managing director of Air New Zealand, and then going to Australia to run the Commonwealth Bank of Australia, taking it from the fifth largest company on the Australian stock exchange to the largest. Now living back in his hometown of Auckland, he currently chairs the boards of Fletcher Building and Contact Energy. What changed his health and lifestyle? The discovery that he actually had Type 1 diabetes.

Initially I was diagnosed as having Type 2 diabetes and I was being treated as a Type 2. With my condition starting to deteriorate, I went to Rick Cutfield, and he looked at me, and said, 'You don't look like a Type 2 candidate,' straight off the bat. 'We'll run a blood antibody test.'

The test came back and indicated that all along I had had a predisposition genetically for Type 1 diabetes. It was one of those cases where something could trigger it, but the problem was not really knowing what that trigger actually was.

When I retired from the ASB Bank back in 2001, I wasn't feeling particularly well at all. At that stage I was still being treated as a Type 2, and so I was feeling pretty unhealthy.

The upshot of all that was that Rick came into the picture on the back of some work that was done in Australia by another specialist. Rick ran the blood antibody test and said, 'You're Type 1 predisposed and I think this is Type 1. It's obvious you need insulin.'

And so I went on insulin. And within a week or two I started to feel amazingly better. That was in the period between me leaving ASB and taking on the job at Air New Zealand. It was about four and a half months between retiring from ASB and going to Air New Zealand.

If you'd told me at the time I left ASB that I'd be working in an executive role four and a half months later, I would have been highly, highly dubious, because I felt so bad, health-wise.

Since then I take four shots of insulin per day at breakfast, lunch and dinner, and then at bedtime.

The injections are virtually painless. Sometimes I hit a nerve, which gives me a little bit of a jab but not as bad as a sting though.

The needles are very short, so they don't penetrate very far, and at the same time they are very, very small in diameter and so therefore they're not particularly invasive.

It does take a little bit of getting used to. I used to inject into the stomach area, which can lead to the creation of a sort of ring of fat, which doesn't look particularly great. I then moved to the thigh, and I find the thigh is much better. It doesn't make any difference to the effectiveness of the insulin but I find it's a much more convenient place to inject.

I've never found it difficult to find a time and space for the injection. I can move myself away somewhere and carry out the injection without anybody realising. Most people I deal with would probably not have any idea that I'm a Type 1 diabetic.

The trick is making sure that you're getting the dosage right, because the last thing you want to end up with is what's called 'hypoglycaemic shock', where you end up with your blood sugar too low. That's when you can risk going into a coma. Balancing the insulin becomes pretty much second nature. If you eat something that's got a high level of carbohydrate, you might need a little bit more insulin.

I think it comes down to the fact that you have to manage the situation, and you have to make yourself reasonably aware of what's happening, why it's happening, and how you can control it. Some people have very poor control of their diabetes because they don't give it the appropriate level of focus and importance. It's not just about taking the injections, and getting your doses right. It's making sure that you're eating well, that you're eating a good balanced diet.

It's also important that you're doing exercise, and I'd have to say that I'm probably healthier today in many respects than I would have been if I hadn't have had diabetes at all, because I'm much more focused on what I eat and on making sure I get exercise. I've got a need to do that, and so it gives me that impetus to make sure that I'm looking after myself, probably better than I would if I was otherwise healthy, and didn't have diabetes.

I don't regard myself as an invalid or anything like that. It's just something I have to live with. I think if you take a positive view of it and think, 'Hey, this is what it is, and I'm not going to let it interfere with my life,' you can get on and live your life well.

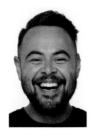

Nickson Clark

Nickson Clark is one of the morning crew on Mai FM in Auckland. He has his dream job, keeps fit at the gym, and plays touch football and league. Nickson today is lean and active. It wasn't always the case. When still in his early 20s, he was diagnosed with Type 2 pre-diabetes.

All through high school I was quite big. I've got a tonne of photos I could show you where I've got no neck; I'm marshmallow man.

When you're a kid, your parents tell you it's just puppy fat and that you'll grow out of it, and you believe that. Then when you start getting to your later teenage years, and you've left secondary school, and you go to uni, and you're still not losing that puppy fat, then it kind of clicks.

I'm half Polynesian. I'm half Samoan and in the Samoan culture it's offensive if you don't eat the food that is presented to you by your family, and if you're not eating a lot, or you're choosing foods that are westernised, you're being disrespectful.

My mum, who is full Samoan, and my grandparents would always dish out the coconut cream and the palusami (a savoury dish where seasoned coconut cream is wrapped in taro leaves and cooked). I was eating all that, and, obviously, if KFC comes onto the table, that too. I'm an only child, too, so I got spoilt in that sense where we could go to McDonald's all the time.

By my early 20s the highest weight I got up to was 120kg. That was the point where I thought I had to do something about it. I didn't know about my pre-diabetic condition at that stage, but I knew that I wasn't healthy. You're breaking out in sweats, and it's winter, and you're like, 'Why am I sweaty?' Or you're getting puffed and out of breath. I knew something was wrong, but I just thought I was fat.

So at 120kg what comes next sounds like a romantic comedy, but it's not. I went through quite a messy break-up and at that point I thought, 'I've got to lose weight, I'm not healthy, I don't feel good.' My relationship fell apart and I thought it was the end of the world.

I thought, 'If I can get myself looking right, I can make her jealous, and she'd want me back.' So I went to the gym and I started to eat what I thought was healthy. But I didn't really know what I was doing. I started to lose weight very quickly. Then I thought, 'I don't feel too well' and I was going to the toilet quite a bit. I was constantly urinating and I thought it wasn't right.

I lost a lot of weight very quickly, I went from 120kg to 66kg in about three months. That's not healthy. You can't maintain that. That's the one thing that I think people really misinterpret. They think these quick-fix diets are going to keep you healthy, and lose weight, but you can't maintain that lifestyle.

I didn't really have my diet under control, although I thought I was making better choices. That's when I had to go to the doctor and find out what was actually going on. They did a few tests and that's when they told me I was pre-diabetic, and I needed to sort out my weight because it was fluctuating as well. That's when it all started for me and I had to get an understanding of what was going on.

So it was about seven years ago when I got diagnosed with pre-diabetes Type 2. Then I got to Type 2 because I was making those bad choices. That was just due to my lifestyle and the bad food choices and lack of exercise.

The only person I told was my dad. My dad is European and he's not an emotional man. He deals with facts and works his way from there. I talked to Dad and said, 'This is what the doctor said. I don't want to freak out Mum but can you help me through this?' My dad is a chef and he helped me.

I talked to the doctor, and they talked to me about a balance of exercise and the foods that I need to stay away from for a little bit. Not opting totally for sugar-free options but just opting for healthier options. Not trying to do anything drastic but just easing back. Less processed, more natural foods.

For a good year I stayed on that and I've been able to balance my weight now. I'm more in control. I was on some medication they gave me. It wasn't insulin but it was just to balance it out.

Ever since then, over the last four or five years, I've been able to maintain a healthy weight. I'm now about 79–80kg. I go to the gym. I used to be all about cardio, but I felt like I had to mix it up so I do CrossFit. I go to Les Mills in the city, and then our local leisure centre in West Auckland as well.

I try to get amongst the group fitness thing. I love group fitness because we get together. A gym can be intimidating, but group fitness is fun. It's quite motivating to see other people on the same journey as yourself. You keep everybody accountable as well, and they're keeping you accountable.

I also play touch and I've played rugby league. Throughout the journey that's definitely been one of the things that's been a positive for me, because you feel good when you're playing sport, and it's like a chain reaction.

One of the reasons I love working with Diabetes New Zealand is because their support system is encouraging people to make changes now before it gets too late. That's what I give them massive props for. I know that that sounds really preachy. It's like 'change your life, change your life' but it's the truth.

It's the hardest thing to try to sell somebody sometimes without being preachy. But with Diabetes New Zealand, they're giving you the tools to make those subtle changes so you don't get worse, or get to a point where you're really bad. Those building blocks are helping us live a better and healthier life.

I've seen that in my own family. My nana has got Type 2 diabetes and thankfully she's been able to make those changes. She's worked through it.

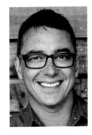

Brett McGregor

Brett McGregor was the deputy-principal of an intermediate school in Christchurch when entering Masterchef *on television in 2006 changed everything. Brett won, and now cooking is his life. He's written three bestselling cookbooks, produces cooking videos, and has made two series of his own show,* Taste of a Traveller. *His passion for healthy eating and living is partly driven by the tragic story of what happened to his closest friend, who had Type 2 diabetes.*

Aaron and I go back to primary school in Taranaki. I went to a school called Marfell Primary and he went to Spotswood Primary. We used to play sports against each other all through primary school. We also played in the same rugby team, Spotswood Old Boys, in New Plymouth.

He was a year older than me and, from the age of about seven or eight, we started to hang out with each other. His parents owned a dairy about a kilometre from my house. His mum still lives there now.

So Aaron and I go way back and we probably started hanging out more and more as we got older. He would have been maybe 11 or 12 when he was diagnosed with Type 2 diabetes. Originally I thought he had diabetes his whole life, but I've done a little bit more investigating and he developed it in his younger years.

He was a true Kiwi bloke. He never really looked after himself that much, I suppose, and lived life to the full. He was always out there, the first one wanting to have a party, that kind of stuff. And then, as he got older, the diabetes became more and more of a problem for him.

He was slightly overweight and I know that he was taking small amounts of insulin when he was younger but his dosage was getting constantly greater as he got older. When he really started to fail to look after himself was when he moved with his partner from New Plymouth up to Auckland.

He would have been about 40 at this stage, and he noticed that he had a little black mark on the top of his foot, and was a little bit feverish. He thought he had the flu, and there was just something else wrong with his foot. He didn't really care too much about it, but then he noticed that the black mark was appearing on the bottom of his foot.

His partner, Michelle, had been telling him, 'Listen mate, just go to the doctor. Go to the doctors. Go and get it checked out.' So he went off to the doctor and that day they said, 'You've got to go straight to hospital, it's bad.' And so they took him to hospital. By this stage, it had been a couple of weeks since he'd noticed the black mark on his foot and his toes were starting to turn black.

When I went and saw him I lifted back the blanket and I just went, 'Oh my God, dude. What are you doing?' He looked like he had frostbite. So I said, 'What's the worst-case scenario?' He said, 'Worst-case scenario, mate, they're going to take half my foot off.' We were pretty freaked out about that. He went into surgery that day, and when he came out they had taken his leg off just below the knee.

He went home for recovery and was starting to get blurred vision. At that stage, they couldn't even get his wheelchair into the house. His flat was just not ready for that kind of stuff. He was just hobbling around.

One day he went to the bathroom and, because his vision was so bad, he fell over and broke the femur in his leg that had been operated on. They couldn't put a cast on it, so they just bandaged it and he went through that pain. He became blind in one eye because of the pressure and then his vision got worse in the other eye.

He was in and out of hospital, as you would imagine. Finally it got so bad he was on dialysis but his body couldn't handle the dialysis and he was having a lot of trouble. It was like they were just keeping him alive sometimes, and then finally his heart gave way and that was it. He was 43 years old.

I've never met anyone like him. His nickname was Buddha. He was a 'give you the shirt off his back' kind of guy, but when it came to himself he couldn't care less. Couldn't care. The last three years of his life with his wife Michelle were just really tough. They really struggled. It destroyed their lives.

It was just crazy that throughout his whole life if he had just made a couple of small changes, maybe didn't do some of the stuff that he was doing, he could have controlled what was happening and maybe turned his life around.

The lesson for me, in the loss we all felt, is that whether it's prostate cancer or diabetes, or whatever it is, you've just got to go, as you get older, and have your medical checks. Just get checked. It's no big deal. I look at my son Jack and I just think about the years that I want to be around for him.

Talk about it with your mates. Let's get it out in the open and stop feeling so, I suppose you'd call it, inhibited about it.

I think blokes these days are getting more open. It's not like my grandfather's generation, but being open about your health is still in its infancy. We need to grow that.

MY FAVOURITE SPORTING JOKE

A golfer in the Waikato hits his ball into the rough. As he's searching for it a little man in green tights and a pointed hat pops up.

'Hey,' says the golfer. 'You must be a leprechaun.'

'I am indeed, sir,' says the little man in a strong Irish accent. 'And I'm not just any leprechaun. I am The Famous Irish Golfing Leprechaun, and this is your lucky day. I'm on holiday in New Zealand, and if you wish I can make you the best golfer in the world.'

'I'd love that,' says the Waikato man. 'Golf is my great passion.'

'I must warn you of one thing,' says the leprechaun. 'There is a price to pay. For every degree your golf improves, your love life suffers. Twice as good a golfer, half as good a love life. Ten times as good a golfer, ten times as bad a love life.'

'I don't care,' says the golfer. 'Make me 100 times better.'

'Jaysus, you realise your love life will be 100 times worse?'

'I love golf. Make me 100 times better.'

The leprechaun snaps his fingers and disappears into the long grass.

The golfer finds the ball, drives to the green, one putts for a birdie, then goes on to smash the course record. Two weeks later he wins his club championship, six weeks later he takes the Waikato provincial title. He goes to Paraparaumu and wins the national amateur championship. Every round he has there lowers the course record.

Just on a year after his meeting with the leprechaun he's in Dublin, red hot favourite to win the world amateur title, with an offer to turn pro and head to the PGA tour already on the table.

On the tee for the first round of the championship his drive, as always now, is over 300 metres. But at the apex a wee gust of wind takes his ball into the rough on the left-hand side.

'No problem,' he thinks. 'One shot to the green, down in one, and it's a birdie to start.'

When he gets to the rough he finds a wee man standing next to his ball. The Famous Irish Golfing Leprechaun.

'Mate, am I glad to see you. Everything you promised with my golf game has come true. I could never thank you enough.'

'Sure, that's grand,' says the leprechaun, 'but could I ask one thing? How's your love life?'

'Not bad.'

'Not bad? One hundred times worse than before and you say it's not bad?'

'Yeah, not bad.'

'If you don't mind me asking, how many times have you made love in the year since we met?'

'About five times.'

'Five times? A good-looking young man like you thinks making love five times in a whole year is not bad?'

'Hey listen, mate,' says the golfer. 'It's not bad for a Catholic priest from Tokoroa.'

Five Great Crime Novels
Worth Hunting Out

Paul Thomas is one of New Zealand's most successful crime novelists. He has written five Tito Ihaka novels, the most recent, Fallout, *was a bestseller in 2015. His other great passion is sport. He writes a weekly column for the* Listener *and has written two biographical books on cricketer John Wright.*

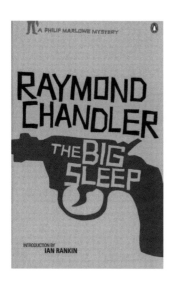

The Big Sleep
by Raymond Chandler (1939)

This is how the first of Chandler's seven Philip Marlowe novels begins: 'It was about 11 o'clock in the morning, mid-October, with the sun not shining and a look of hard, wet rain in the clearness of the foothills. I was wearing my powder blue suit, with a dark-blue shirt, tie and display handkerchief, black brogues, dark blue socks with blue clocks on them. I was neat, clean, shaved and sober, and I didn't care who knew it. I was calling on four million dollars.'

Chandler's influence on popular culture was immense. He revolutionised crime fiction while, as *Time* magazine put it, 'inspiring more poses and parodies than any other writer of the [20th] century save Hemingway'.

Out went the formal mystery novel — predominantly British, plot-driven, law-abiding, middle-class; in came the realistic crime novel — predominantly American, character-driven, extra-legal, uncouthly democratic. Freed from constraints, crime fiction could tackle themes and subjects that had previously been the domain of social realist novelists and did so with a gusto, fluency and narrative drive incompatible with high-brow literature.

Chandler also created a literary archetype who succeeded the tamers of the Wild West in the popular imagination: the wise-cracking private eye with a .38 Special and a fifth of Scotch in his bottom drawer and a powerfully evocative voice — cynical, world-weary, crackling with cussedness and self-contempt, yet with a persistent throb of bruised romanticism.

In what may well be the finest tribute one great writer has paid another, his successor Ross Macdonald (see below) said Chandler 'wrote like a slumming angel and invested the sun-blinded streets of Los Angeles with a romantic presence'.

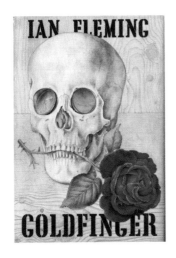

Goldfinger
by Ian Fleming (1959)

Despite the James Bond books' vast commercial success and socio-cultural impact, they're now essentially pop culture artefacts. That's a pity because the best of them are classics of the genre and Fleming is a much under-rated writer. He wasn't a great plotter and the dialogue is almost exclusively expositional, but he was very good at colour and wrote great set pieces.

Like the golf game in this book. Having got under Auric Goldfinger's skin by catching him cheating at two handed canasta, Bond gives the cad another comeuppance over 18 holes. The fictional

Royal St Mark's course is based on Royal St George's at Sandwich, Kent, where in 1964, aged 56, Fleming ate lunch for the very last time.

An added benefit of reading Bond is that, no matter how much you drink, he drinks way more than you do. Before a night of high-stakes gambling in *Casino Royale*, Bond puts away the following. Pre-lunch: an Americano (Campari and sweet vermouth); with lunch: a couple of Scotches; pre-dinner: a dry martini comprising three parts gin, one part vodka and one part vermouth; with dinner: a small carafe of vodka and a bottle of champagne (shared); post-dinner: three bottles of champagne.

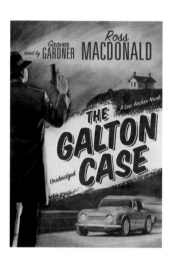

The Galton Case
by Ross Macdonald (1959)

Although regarded by crime-fiction buffs and cultural studies scholars as one of the holy trinity of American crime writing (along with Chandler and Dashiell Hammett), Macdonald never enjoyed the others' name recognition. His real name was Kenneth Millar. Having adopted a nom de plume to avoid confusion with his mystery writer wife Margaret Millar, he spent the rest of his career being mistaken for another American crime novelist, John D. Macdonald.

The Library of America is now republishing a dozen of Macdonald's Lew Archer novels, including this one in which he shakes off the Chandler influence and finds his own voice. When you compare their respective bodies of work, there's little doubt that, while Chandler blazed the trail, Macdonald is the superior novelist.

He may also be the only writer to whom a rock album has been dedicated: Warren Zevon's *Bad Luck Streak in Dancing School*.

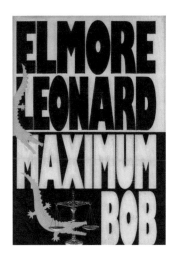

Maximum Bob
by Elmore Leonard (1991)

Martin Amis had this to say about Elmore Leonard: 'His characters are equipped not with obligingly suggestive childhoods or case histories, but with a cranial jukebox of situation comedies, talk shows and advertising jingles, their dreams and dreads all mediated and second-hand. They are not lost souls or dead souls. Terrible and pitiable (and often downright endearing), they are simply junk souls: quarter pounders, with cheese.'

Sound familiar? Arguably without Leonard, there would have been no *Pulp Fiction*. And without *Pulp Fiction*, we wouldn't have had the avalanche of literary and cinematic sub-Tarantino imitations, knock-offs and homages that continue to this day. Up to you whether that would have been a good or bad thing.

(Quentin Tarantino turned Leonard's novel *Rum Punch* into the movie *Jackie Brown*; Steven Soderbergh's *Out of Sight* and Barry Sonnenfeld's *Get Shorty* are other standouts amongst the many screen adaptations of Leonard's work. The wonderful TV series *Justified* is based on a Leonard short story and features his recurring character, US Marshal Raylan Givens.)

'Maximum Bob' is the nickname of a right-wing Floridian judge who invariably imposes the maximum sentence for minimal offences. It's typical Leonard: dense, intricate, funny, totally convincing yet apparently effortless. In writing as in sport, the greats make it look easy.

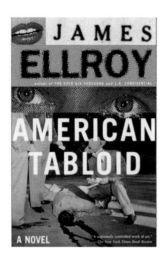

American Tabloid
by James Ellroy (1995)

The self-described 'demon dog' (or sometimes 'foul owl') of crime writing, Ellroy works on the premise that America has two histories: the official one and the secret one. His mission in life is to shine a light on the secret one. It's fitting that this, his greatest work, should revolve around the assassination of John Kennedy, the wellspring for much of the paranoia and conspiracism that has undermined public trust in America's political class and institutions of state in the decades since.

I once observed Ellroy introduce himself to an Australian literary gathering with a shout-out to the 'panty sniffers and kangaroo fuckers' in the audience. Later, in private, he admitted the demented, far right, demon dog persona is a marketing tool; he is, in fact, an understated, liberal-minded teetotaller.

Breakups
Just the Facts

There are studies suggesting that, after the death of a loved one, the most difficult thing to deal with emotionally in your life is a divorce. Many men and women find themselves stunned when a marriage or long-term relationship ends, struggling to deal with the upheaval (especially if there are children involved), and if it happens to you then you may find yourself battling to make clear, sensible decisions.

The fence at the top of the cliff for a relationship that's in major trouble is counselling. It doesn't need to be a hugely expensive experience. A good place to seek help is at a Citizens Advice Bureau. You can check for a bureau in your area by going to their website: cab.org.nz.

Hopefully your relationship can be repaired. But the harsh reality is that about one in three marriages will not last forever. Figures from Statistics New Zealand show that one-third of people married in 1980 were divorced before they reached their silver, 25th wedding anniversary.

If, despite all best efforts, your relationship has come to an end, there will be emotional costs. But there are also, at a time when everyone is likely to be feeling fragile, some practical issues to be dealt with.

What should you know about what follows? Here are some answers to nine questions that are likely to arise.

What if you both want a divorce?

If you and your partner in a marriage (or civil union) agree the marriage is over, all that is required is to file for what is now officially called a dissolution of marriage or civil union and, from the time your application is filed, it is unlikely to be more than a month before the dissolution is granted.

What if your partner refuses a divorce?

In a less enlightened age a divorce could only be forced on a partner who wanted to stay married with proof of unfaithfulness. A high-selling national newspaper called *Truth* used to run a page of shame, a treasure trove for gossips, which listed that week's divorces, and named the third party involved in sexual affairs.

Now the only grounds for the dissolution of a marriage is that the marriage has broken down irreconcilably, and that's defined by law as the fact that you've been living apart for two years.

Judge Laurence Ryan is the head of the Family Court in New Zealand. He says, 'You don't have to prove adultery, you don't have to prove anything about the other person. You only have to prove that you've been apart for two years.

'You can do it on your own. The other person can try to say there's still a chance the marriage will work, but that isn't a defence to stop the dissolution. For example, some people may have religious beliefs that make them strongly opposed to the idea of divorce, and they won't agree to it.

'So sometimes you have to go through court. If you've been apart for two years, the judge will have to ultimately say, "I'm sorry, but even if this person won't go to counselling, or that he or she won't make an effort to stay in the marriage, that's not a defence."'

What about de facto relationships?

What is your legal situation if you and your partner have never married, or been in a civil union, but have lived together in a de facto (a Latin expression that means 'in reality') relationship, basically a marriage in all but name?

In most cases, only people who have lived together in a de facto relationship for at least three years are covered unless there is a child involved.

The court will look at many things when deciding whether two people are in a de facto relationship, including:

- how long the relationship lasted
- their care and support of children
- the extent to which the couple share a home
- whether they have a sexual relationship
- their financial and property arrangements and how much they depend on each other
- their ownership, use and purchase of property
- how committed they've both been to a shared life
- who does the housework and other household duties
- if the partners are known to family and friends or other people as a couple.

What should you do to protect yourself legally?

Whether you are leaving a marriage, civil union or de facto relationship, find a specialist family lawyer, if possible. 'You wouldn't,' as a senior lawyer once told me, 'go to your GP for an operation.' To find that family lawyer, someone who knows what pitfalls to avoid, and what to do that's right, a good place to start would be the website justice. govt.nz/family.

Once you've found an experienced lawyer, be sensible and follow his or her advice. 'Most senior family lawyers have been there and done that,' says Judge Ryan. 'They appear in court, and they can advise you of the likely outcome if there are disputes.'

What's likely to happen to a house and money?

The courts in New Zealand see marriage, civil unions or de facto relationships as an equal partnership, and so both assets and liabilities are shared equally. In other words, if a court makes a decision, you and your former partner will get half each.

'The way we look at it,' says Judge Ryan, 'is that nobody loses anything. Together you've accumulated that wealth and you divide the assets equally at the end. The basic principle is that everything is equal.

'Exceptions do come in. If you and your wife have young children that need a roof over their head, it's likely she will be able to persuade a judge to let her and the children live in the house for a period. In that case, you're not going to get your hands on your share of the house for a while. That's a possibility.'

What specifically happens when a dissolution is granted?

If the dissolution is not contested, you won't even see a judge. A Family Court registrar (a civil servant who oversees the day-to-day running of the Court) will grant it. In an uncontested divorce you don't even have to go into a courtroom after papers are filed.

If things turn nasty, how do you get to see your children?

'As Family Court judges, we see a tiny percentage of couples that are warring,' says Judge Ryan. 'Most people in marriages or relationships can, and do, sort out their relationships with their kids without coming anywhere near a court. We see, therefore, the tip of the iceberg and the most difficult cases. We see the worst of it.

'A lot of the people we see are using the children as weapons, and it's to attack the other. "You left me for my best friend, don't think I'm going to allow my children to be near her. So you're not going to be able to take the children to stay at your house if she's there."

'The children just want their parents to be happy. Initially they want them to remain together, of course. Even if it's been horrific they want them to be together. So yes, people use them as weapons, but it's a very small group.

'They need professional assistance and the sooner the better. What people do is get entrenched in positions and they start fighting. So the sooner you can get in there with some therapy, the sooner you can get them to sit down and talk and see that the children have to be the focus, not the other person, the better.'

If things can't be resolved in a fair and reasonable way, to have what is legally known as care and contact, aka visiting rights, you need to apply to the Family Court.

What's the Family Court like?

Not remotely like the movie *A Few Good Men*, when Tom Cruise and Jack Nicholson snarl at each other until Nicholson snaps and let's a guilty cat out of the bag. The emotions may be just as raw, but the aim of the judges in a Family Court is to be as civilised and fair as possible.

The Family Court is a civil court, not as formal as a criminal court. After all, no criminals are involved, just normal people who can hopefully make the best of a sad situation. There are no spectators, no reporters. It's nobody's business but your own.

Recent law reforms mean that fewer and fewer people in Family Court are represented by a lawyer.

A small ray of light is that the judge hearing the case will almost certainly be sympathetic to the fact you're very nervous. Family Court judges have special training to make sure someone without a lawyer gets treated fairly.

'We're all very respectful of people who do not have a lawyer,' says Judge Ryan. 'We do understand that they often don't have much of a choice.

'Most judges will bend over backwards to explain how it works. They'll say, "This is where you give evidence," and explain what the order of proceedings is. "After you've given your evidence your wife's lawyer will ask questions, and you can fill in gaps at the end. After your wife has given evidence you'll be able to ask questions."'

How hard is it to give evidence?

Remember, if the day comes when you have to give evidence in a Family Court, you are not going into a hostile environment. Judge Ryan himself, who worked in courtrooms for many years as a lawyer before he became a judge, is very mindful of how nerve-wracking a witness box can be for the man in the street.

Not long after he was appointed a judge, he had to appear as a witness in a trial by jury. 'I felt quite intimidated as a witness. Standing in the witness box and looking at a jury takes you a long way out of your comfort zone.'

Judge Ryan agrees entirely with the enormously helpful and comforting advice a highly experienced lawyer gave to actor Laurie Dee and I when we successfully sued Television New Zealand for a breach of contract in the 1980s over scriptwriting we had done for *The Billy T James Show*.

When we gave our evidence, the lawyer told us, 'Don't even think about lying, and, if you don't have a clear memory about something, just be honest and say you can't remember. Don't say anything unless you're quite sure about it. If you do that, you'll never go wrong in a courtroom.'

Finally, remember that good behaviour does get rewarded

If you're a father, the more fairly and decently you behave after your marriage or relationship breaks up, the more likely you are to have a warm and good relationship with your children in the years ahead.

The Magic of Music

Mike Chunn and music are soulmates. While still at Sacred Heart boarding school in Auckland, known to family and the school as Jonathon Chunn, he bonded with a boy from Te Awamutu called Brian Finn. They started using the first names Mike and Tim and, by the early 1970s, had founded a band they called Split Ends. Renamed Split Enz, the band took them around the world but Mike eventually chose to settle back in Auckland. He had success again, playing sold-out concerts and making the charts with his brother Geoff in Citizen Band. He then ran the Mushroom record label, signing DD Smash and the Dance Exponents, and later headed APRA, the organisation that makes sure songwriters get their royalties. His passion for music is now channelled into the Play It Strange Trust, dedicated to finding songwriters in New Zealand schools. Music is, he says, a joy, not to mention a comfort, and here he shares those feelings.

If we could see songs they would be luminous trails in the breath of space. And from there they drift down upon us and we absorb them. And we respond emotionally to every one we hear. Some lodge themselves in our hearts where they reside until we take our last breath. Such songs have their own special purpose. The American playwright Ben Hecht put it well: 'Old songs are more than tunes; they are little houses in which our hearts once lived.'

There's the rub . . . an unimportant factor. Either they live in our hearts or our hearts live in them. No matter. It's a deeply symbiotic union and we have them there, always, to save us; to draw us away from the dark.

If we can go back in time . . .

I didn't think about it then, although my subconscious must have been reeling. One day, at the age of 13 I'm sitting on the back deck of the family home in Otahuhu watching V-shaped flocks of birds, all in their perfect formation, drifting to the east. (Were they lost? I thought birds flew north.) My mother's comforting call — 'Dinner's ready!'

I say that but that's not how it happened. She would ring a bell but to put that in here verbatim might leave you wondering. How would it sit? *Dong dong dong dong.* But let's move on.

The next day I'm lying in a bed in a dormitory with about 40 other boys my age. I look around. The ceiling is very high. We all have pyjamas that pretty much look the same. A song is playing on the old wooden radio.

The next evening I'm back there again. Looking around. My hands are stinging from being caned for talking to a young lad whose name still rests with me as part of the record. Bernard. I spoke to him in night study class. I don't know what I said to him.

But what rises above all this *stuff* — that turns stinging flesh and a deep desire to run away into a subdued *whatever* — is what I am hearing again. We are in February 1966 and a valve radio high up on a shelf in the dormitory is on — it was on each night in the lead-up to lights-out largesse (excuse me, I thought I'd try some alliteration) — and a record called 'We Can Work It Out' by The Beatles is being broadcast in all its muddy AM manner and I am mesmerised. Truly and utterly absorbed. The radio is turned off and the lights are turned out. And the song remains. And I feel happy. I turn it over in my mind. In my mind's eye, I am a Beatle.

The next night it is the same. The lights go out. And the song remains.

To this day — if the detail of life subsides into some gargoyled, rococo obstruction, I can click a mouse, maybe push a 'play' — something — to bring that song back to life. But really, I'm allowing it to burst from my heart and sing to me. And carry me away from dross, turmoil, demands and emptiness. Flying. And I feel better. I feel elevated. This is the truth.

Each of you reading this will have the same scenario. A song that pushes away whatever is driving you mad. I have a number of them now; all taking their place, happily in waiting.

At the age of 63, I have had the pleasure of growing old at the same steady pace as Bob Dylan. While he is about 10 years older than me, it is the way he carries time with him in his records that enthrals me. We grow old together. He sings to me about me. And I am a better man. Whether it is the revelation of flaws, points of difference or matters of romance and the union of people. That's okay. I want him to tell me about it all. That is an important part of songs and their deep attachment. Are we learning from them?

Dylan's album *Oh Mercy* was when I first felt this man walking beside me, talking in my ear. It was London and Margaret Thatcher was in tow. I had my Aiwa portable cassette player with me with my Sony Professional Walkman headphones after hopping off a double-decker bus near Green Arbour Court. Alight in EC1. The big, lonely city. The *Sun* newspaper poster of the day featured a huge headline 'Up Yours Delors'. The sub-heading '. . . Sun readers are urged to tell the French fool where to stuff his ECU'.

His Royal Bobness sings away: 'We live in a political world; Where mercy walks the plank . . .' By the end of the song I'm seeing things in a different light. A clear vision.

Every country brings songwriters like Bob Dylan into their multiple structures, strictures, points of order and pictures (dig that rhyme). Canada with its beautiful mix of English and French finds true inspiration in their top-flight songwriters. You can't go past Joni Mitchell; especially in her Reprise label years. What really matters is that she brings a unique turn on everyday life in its universality.

When she sings: 'Woke up, it was a Chelsea morning, and the first thing that I heard; Was a song outside my window, and the traffic wrote the words.'

Joy.

No need to wake up and think, 'Ah the grind. The same old pointless exercise of pursuit of vague yadda yadda and mumble grumble.' Play some Joni and be happy. She is talking about us.

Or let's keep it in here. Lil ole New Zealand. In the suburban streets of Te Aroha, Geraldine or Hawera. And the rest. You've just dropped into a petrol station to buy some petrol. It's early morning. You think, 'Some lucky bastards are still lying in bed.' You wonder about wandering away. You don't. What to do? Play Don McGlashan's 'Lucky Stars'.

Henderson Park is still in the dark
And I stop to put gas in the car
I stand in line behind a barefoot man
Who's buying cigarettes and a chocolate bar
I catch sight of my reflection in the smash-proof glass
And I thank my Lucky Stars

You will cruise off down the road with a smile on your face. A song has befriended you and placed you in a warm perspective; a gentle purpose.

The power of a song. There will be times when you play them again and again. The more the better. And again. And you keep that smile on your face. The power of a song.

In the end, it is the subconscious that ensures songs maintain their healing presence. We may not think about them, we may not analyse them or submit them to debate. But those that play an important part in our life, at any age, maintain our equilibrium and steer us in the right direction. They rise to the surface like the morning sun.

Our son was five years old when I used to play the soundtrack to the movie *The Harder They Come* — Jamaican reggae and ska tunes with a cool mix of celebration, menace and community. Johnny would sit at the table eating porridge or cereal quietly listening. I played that album every morning for about a year. And then I moved on to the Nick Drake album *Bryter Layter*.

About two years later we were living in another house and one evening I put *The Harder They Come* album on and it played away. At exactly the same moment, Johnny was given his evening meal of chicken and an array of vegetables. He sat there for some time just staring at the plate and listening to the songs. After a while he said, 'This is a weird-looking breakfast.'

The power of song.

Testicular Cancer
Looking After the Boys

As men, we have a lot of nicknames for our testicles. Nuts, balls, the boys, the apricots, bollocks, the Crown jewels, the plums, the goolies. So far, so relaxed. But you'll never hear us brag about their size. Or their attractiveness. No woman has ever had to reassure an anxious bed partner that his testicles were big enough.

Which might explain why, with testicular cancer, some guys will literally allow themselves to die of embarrassment, because they can't stand the thought of a doctor looking at their nuts. The really crazy thing is that although testicular cancer is often very aggressive, it's also a cancer where early treatment has a massive success rate.

And guess what? You can be the one who privately first checks for any signs of problems. At what age should you be checking? At any time in your life from the time you reach puberty.

Many of us think of testicular cancer as a young man's disease but, while cases of it in a very young man are the saddest stories, it's not true they're the only ones. From the time your voice drops a basic check will always be worthwhile.

So how should you check, whatever your age? It's literally as simple as being in the shower and running your hand over your scrotum and giving each nut a squeeze. As a man, you know I don't need to add to only squeeze gently.

'If you check them in the shower, and there is a lump, you should feel it reasonably early on. It might be the size of a pea to start with,' says urological surgeon Jim Duthie.

If you do find a lump, summon up your courage and take yourself, and your testicles, to a doctor.

If you're a teenager reading this, please listen up. Or if you have a teenage son, or grandson, and the idea of talking with him about him handling his testicles feels more painful than sticking needles in your eyes, maybe just hand him the book, ask him to read this chapter, and then leave the room. Because it's staggering how far teenagers will let a problem with their testicles develop before they'll do anything.

Jim Duthie says he and his urologist colleagues all have a true story about an 18- or 19-year-old who comes to see them with a tumour the size of a grapefruit on a testicle. Let me say that again. The size of a grapefruit.

It's an unfortunate fact that some guys, at any age, not just teenagers, get spooked when a medical problem occurs in the groin area.

'Older guys who have trouble with their waterworks,' says Jim, 'who are worried about prostate cancer, often start off deluding themselves and saying, "Well, you know, it's probably nothing. Probably just a bit of infection; it'll settle down." And every day the problem's getting bigger, and they're just getting more and more worried about it, more and more sick about the idea of dying, and they don't see anybody about it.'

Thinking 'it'll be fine, I hope' about your prostate is as silly as taking the same attitude to testicular cancer. Why is it so worthwhile to get lumps on your testicles checked quickly? Because if you do, two things will happen, and both will see you leading a happy life for years to come.

'First off the bat,' says Jim, 'not everybody's got cancer. You can just have lumpy nuts. There's all sorts of plumbing down there. If you've had a vasectomy, and if you are examined down there thoroughly enough, in behind the nut, you will often find a little nodule there. And that is just par for the course after a vasectomy. All along that plumbing work, you can get little cysts that are completely benign.'

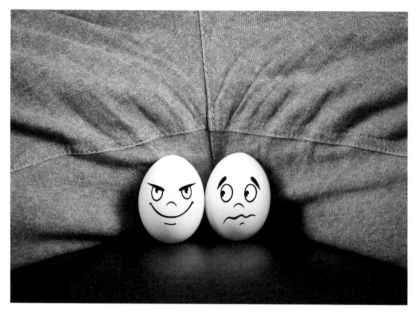

If they feel a little strange, have the boys checked by a doctor.

In the harmless cyst case you've taken a major stress out of your life. But what if the lump isn't benign?

'This is often an aggressive cancer, but the good news is that it almost always responds to treatment. It is almost always curable, even when it spreads. But the sooner you get to it, the simpler the treatment is, so that's why it's worthwhile seeing a doctor as soon as you notice something in the shower. If it's in the early stages, we remove the testicle and that can be the end of it.'

Hang on. Back up the truck right there. Take out the testicle? It's not the big deal it sounds.

'In terms of getting through the operation, it's almost always easy,' says Jim Duthie. 'A fit young guy is in and out of the hospital on the same day, in terms of removing the testicle.'

Losing a testicle has no real side effects. You won't be singing in the Vienna Boys' Choir, losing muscle mass, or eyeing your partner's dresses with envy.

In the case of an older man, someone in his 70s, the cancer's likely to be less aggressive. If the cancer is only in the testicle, surgery alone may be enough. Even if the cancer has spread to other parts of the body, science has developed treatment that has improved your odds of survival enormously.

'The thing that absolutely revolutionised treatment was that in the 1970s they came up with platinum-based chemotherapy for it. It used to be that if you had cancer that had spread beyond the testicle itself, they could do relatively ineffective radiation treatment through your abdomen. If it came back after that you were buggered. But now, even the guys like Lance Armstrong, who had a tumour in his brain, can recover fully. It's an extremely chemotherapy-sensitive type of tumour, and treatment outcomes are very positive.'

Jim has heard first-hand how dramatic the results of chemotherapy treatment for testicular cancer can be. A few years ago he was working in Melbourne, with a Canadian surgeon, who is now one of the doyens of advanced surgery for testicular cancers. He told Jim that back in the 1970s, while the Canadian was working in his own homeland, he had a patient in his 20s who was dying of testicular cancer. There was little to be done, but then the surgeon went to the United States to a fellowship at a hospital where they were experimenting with what was then the new chemotherapy. Amazed at what he saw, he got in touch with his old hospital in Canada, and got the young patient the new treatment.

'Quite soon the patient was discharged from hospital,' says Jim. 'This was back in the 1970s. Five years ago the Canadian surgeon took out that patient's prostate. That's how good the chemo had been at prolonging life.'

Although the inflammation associated with having a tumour in a testicle will often mean its sperm become infertile, if you're a younger man, looking to have, or to complete, a family, all is far from lost. If you're at risk of losing fertility altogether, as can happen with chemotherapy, it's possible to do sperm banking for later use.

For a prime example of how effective treatment in this country is now, consider the story of All Black Aaron Cruden. In 2007 Aaron was an 18-year-old who had completed his first club season out of Palmerston North Boys' High School. Dave Rennie, the coach of the Manawatu Turbos, then sat him down and delivered the sort of message every aspiring young player would love to hear. 'I think if you put in a lot of hard work you can really make a career out of this.'

By the winter of 2008 Aaron was living a young footy player's dream, playing for Rennie's Turbos and making a powerful initial impression. Six games into the rep season everything changed. He was diagnosed with testicular cancer.

'I was quite lucky,' he told me in 2013, 'that mine was caught relatively early, and I had my left testicle removed. But it had spread to the lungs and that's why I had to have some chemotherapy. The doctors were really positive that with a high dose of chemotherapy they could kill it at the source, and that was what they did.

'While I was in hospital it [the chemotherapy] was pretty brutal and tiring. My treatment was nine weeks, broken into three-week cycles. The first week I was in hospital on a drip, getting treatment 24/7, then for the next two weeks I was able to be at home, but I was going in each day for a dose of chemo.

'We repeated that cycle three times. By the third cycle I was pretty drained. But I rebounded pretty quickly, and I really believe that I'm fortunate I was able to do so. I did probably push myself a little bit too hard too early. There were days I woke up very lethargic.

'I still had a couple of months to prove my fitness to Renns [Dave Rennie was now the coach of the New Zealand under-20 side for the world tournament in Japan, scheduled just 10 months after Aaron was diagnosed with cancer] and the coaches, and I was lucky enough to be able to do that.

'When I came into the under-20 squad all the boys were great. They didn't look at me or treat me any differently, and I think that's all people going through that situation want in the end.'

Aaron led his side to a magnificent tournament victory. In the

44–28 win in the final against England he scored two tries, and kicked three conversions and a penalty. 'His performance in the final was just mind-boggling,' says Rennie. 'I'm not sure we'd have won it without him to be honest.'

In the eight years since his cancer was found, his career, with the Chiefs and the All Blacks, has continued to thrive. On a personal level he says, 'I don't think I took things for granted before, but when you go through something life-changing like that you know what is truly important, and you make the most of those opportunities when they arise. Overall I think it's been a good thing for me as a person.'

If, like Aaron, you have a lump on a testicle, fully diagnosing it will be simple and pain-free.

'Ultrasound scanning,' says Jim Duthie, 'is the best thing we've got for looking at the testicular cancers. It's easy, not that hard to get one done in New Zealand, and it's quick and usually painless. So that will almost always give you the definitive answer. We also get a few blood tests if we're particularly suspicious. If the ultrasound shows that it is cancer, you are going to need some blood tests, because some of the tumours make specific chemicals.'

Please don't try to self-diagnose any further than finding a lump. A weird, dangerous theory has made the rounds on social media that if you pee on a pregnancy test stick and it reads positive, you've got cancer.

'Some of the cancers, less than half actually, make beta hCG, which is the chemical that the pregnancy test for women picks up,' says Jim. 'So if you have a lump, a negative test from peeing on a dipstick shouldn't reassure you that you don't have cancer.'

Getting back to treatment. Surgery to remove a tumour may be enough. If not, you'll probably be treated with chemotherapy. It's highly unlikely you'll be treated with radiotherapy. 'It's just not as good as chemotherapy, and is hardly used now,' says Jim Duthie.

After surgery there'll be more scanning. That's to make sure your lymph nodes aren't enlarged. Lymph nodes are found throughout your body and, without going into details only someone with a medical degree could understand, they're part of your immune system. Cancer can enlarge or inflame them and, in very simple terms, cancer can spread from lymph node to lymph node through the body.

'Testicular cancer progresses in a very logical fashion,' says Jim. 'We're lucky we know exactly which lymph nodes get involved first, where they're going to go. So we can look at the scan in the abdomen, and if those lymph glands look fine then you might well be suitable just to have surveillance and then there will be more scans, and more blood tests going forward, but no extra treatment.

'If there's a high risk of it coming back, your oncologist will talk to you about what you want to do, and there's all sorts of things that go into this decision. If you're committed to showing up to all your appointments for the next few years, there's an 80% chance you won't even need any extra treatment. If you need treatment, that treatment cuts the risk of it coming back almost to zero.'

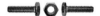

Testicular.org.nz is a website that not only gives informed medical advice, but also has a laugh-out-loud instructional video in which Jim Duthie and another surgeon, Liam Wilson, show how to examine your testicles. Don't be concerned, they use stunt feijoas to illustrate the procedure.

Bloke Paradise

It's been said that within every happy man there's a boy who gets the chance to come out and run around at regular intervals. Luckily you're living in the adventure capital of the world. New Zealand's a country where you can hike, climb, bike, surf, ski or snowboard. Most of the thrills are free and, even if they cost, the charge is usually a lot less than in many other parts of the world. We all know of jet-boating, rafting, and bungee-jumping, which are certainly exciting. But here are a few ways to indulge your inner thrill seeker you may not be so familiar with.

Go black water rafting

Imagine the biggest hose you've ever seen, and it's made of solid rock, 100 metres under ground. Pump water through that hose. Then put on a wetsuit and jump into the foaming stream. That's basically what happens when you go black water rafting at Waitomo. All Blacks fitness trainer Nic Gill says it's the first place he recommends to friends visiting from overseas. 'It's just exhilarating.' Down the road there's the gentle, quiet charms of the Waitomo caves, the ones that have been one of the country's great tourist attractions since 1904. In 1987 a new cave, Ruakuri, was opened. Ruakuri contains a series of chambers, which narrow down at one point to a boiling tube, which can only be traversed by floating on your back, the rock roof less than a metre above, a small waterfall, with a pool deep enough to jump into at its base, and then a high domed grotto, where the stream widens and slows, the rushing noise dies down, and millions of glow-worms light the ceiling. You can check out Black Water Rafting at waitomo.com/black-water-rafting. The original tour is called the Black Labyrinth and costs $138.

Fly like Richie McCaw

Gliding is as close as man will ever get to the pure sensation of flight. Just as a hawk uses the wind to cruise, swoop and dip over the landscape, so a glider pilot reads the thermal winds that eddy over the landscape to keep his fragile but beautiful machine airborne. Richie McCaw fell in love with flight while piloting gliders from Omarama, in Central Otago, a Waitaki District town considered one of the world's great gliding spots. He says, '[In gliding] sometimes fate throws you a curve ball. You have to deal with it the best way you can, survive it, then learn what you can from it.' You can soar with a pilot for 30 minutes over the lakes and mountains that surround the Omarama airfield for $345. And, if you really want the full blast, then for $745 a pilot will take you into the Southern Alps, and, if wind conditions are right, you may even reach the Holy Grail of Kiwi gliding, Aoraki/Mt Cook. To find more details, go to glideomarama.com.

Rocket down the highway

Settle into a McLaren 650S, $700,000 worth of earth-bound rocket. Behind you sits a finely tuned 3.8L, twin turbo-charged V8 motor, the 651hp grunt it delivers gently vibrating your black leather passenger seat. Your professional driver eases down a ramp onto the 4.1km track at Highlands Motorsport Park on the outskirts of Cromwell. The driver pauses and then the powerful supercar leaps forwards, screaming up to 100km/h in three seconds. There are moments on the circuit where the McLaren will top 250km/h. If there's a trace of the petrol head in your being, the McLaren lap is just one of a series of adventures at Highlands, from self-driving go-karts to a single-seater Radical SR3. The cost for the McLaren experience is $169. For more details go to highlands.co.nz.

Walk like a mohawk

If you're a certain age you may remember seeing in an old book photos of Mohawk Indians walking without harnesses on steel beams as they built the Empire State Building in New York. They became known as Skywalkers, for their fearlessness of heights. You don't have to take any risks, but can capture some of that feeling in Auckland, on a harbour bridge walk. Run by AJ Hackett Bungy, the walk takes about 90 minutes and is carefully guided all the way. At one point, you'll be right beside the traffic lanes. 'The biggest buzz,' author Justin Brown told me, 'is walking up a caged staircase which sits metres from vehicles travelling at 80km/h. Metres from trucks which make the bridge actually *move*.' You also get an amazing 360-degree view from the very top of the middle span, 64 metres above the harbour. And if the walk's not quite enough of a buzz for the day, you can add in a bungy jump from a special pod under the bridge. The website is bungy.co.nz/auckland-bridge/auckland-bridge-climb. The cost of the walk is $125. You can add a bungy jump for another $105.

Explore your inner Sir Ed

The whole of the South Island's West Coast should really qualify as a world heritage park. Amongst the diamonds is the Fox Glacier, and for the Coast adventure of your life, the Fox Heli-Hike is the one. It starts in a six-seater Squirrel helicopter, climbing up to 6000ft, giving you a bird's-eye view of Aoraki/Mt Cook and Mt Tasman. This is the territory where Sir Edmund Hillary cut his mountain-climbing teeth before he headed for Mt Everest. Then you'll land on Victoria Flat on the upper levels of the glacier, strap crampons on your feet, and spend hours exploring the glacier. Yes, you'll need to be fit, and have a bit of a head for heights. Your guide will be fully qualified, and can offer you, depending on conditions, the chance to climb up ice walls or abseil down them. You might be lowered into a moulin, a deep ice hole, or shown how to climb an ice pitch using an ice axe and your crampons. You'll wash down lunch with water from the glacier, as pure as any water in the world. For the eight- to nine-hour trip the cost is $650. foxguides.co.nz/extreme-fox-all-day-heli-hike-adventure

Sleep Apnoea
Not Just Snoring

It starts with snoring. At first it's kind of a joke. The joke starts to wear a bit thin when you struggle to stay awake. At meetings, watching TV, or even while driving a car.

At that stage, there's a very good chance you've got a condition called sleep apnoea. (It's pronounced 'app-knee-ah' and it's from the Greek word 'apnoia' or absence of respiration.) It's not uncommon. It picks on men twice as much as it does on women, especially if you're over 50.

Because someone with sleep apnoea can be dismissed as just a loud snorer, it often goes untreated. But there are some pretty serious health risks involved. It can increase your risk of everything from high blood pressure, to stroke, to diabetes, to increasing weight, to liver problems.

So what exactly is sleep apnoea? It involves your tongue being sucked back against the back of the throat to obstruct it for more than 10 seconds, which is about three or four breaths that you can't get in.

'One of the misconceptions,' says Alex Bartle, a doctor who has researched and studied sleep medicine overseas and founded the New Zealand Sleep Well Clinic in 2000, 'is that it's to do with your nose. But it's not, it's a throat problem. It's almost always associated with snoring which is a vibration at the back of your throat.'

Alex says there are three basic signs you may have sleep apnoea.

'One is partner disturbance, or partner rapport, from loud snoring. If somebody snores loudly and persistently they almost certainly have some sleep apnoea. If you're checking on snoring, it's hopeless asking the person, they will nearly always deny it.

'The second thing is waking unrefreshed, waking feeling tired, and then having excessive daytime sleepiness, just feeling tired during the day.

'Rather than putting it down to age and family and work, if it's getting worse and you're snoring a lot then it could be sleep apnoea. That constant tiredness in a loud snorer can lead to what we call cardiac metabolic risk. So if you've got a loud snorer who's tired during the day, and has been diagnosed with, in particular, hypertension, early signs of diabetes, or diabetes, or high blood pressure, then sleep apnoea needs to be considered as a factor.

'Some of the symptoms for cardiac metabolic risk can include getting up a lot to go to the toilet in the night, which you might think was a prostate problem, but is often linked with sleep apnoea.'

There can also be a loss of testosterone production. Among good things that happen when you sleep well is that your body produces testosterone. With sleep apnoea levels of testosterone go down, and very often so does your sex drive.

Who's most likely to get sleep apnoea? If you're an overweight, middle-aged man you're probably at the top of the list. And, if you're a big Maori or Pacific Island guy, with a wide neck, then you're up to three times as likely to get it than a slender white male. But it can also strike lanky people, with a narrow face and a biggish tongue, who are not overweight at all.

(If you're a parent and your child snores, a small number, around 3%, of children up to the age of 12, can have sleep apnoea, almost always caused by enlarged tonsils. If a child's enlarged tonsils are taken out, the success rate for stopping sleep apnoea is 73%.)

If you suspect you might have adult sleep apnoea, your first stop should be with your GP. Alex has a tip for that visit. 'Your doctor will know what sleep apnoea is, but it may not necessarily be on his or her radar. If you go and say, "Look, I'm really tired and I'm not sleeping well", you may end up with sleeping tablets. The idea, of course, is to get you to sleep better, but it often makes sleep apnoea worse. You need to go with specific details about what is going on. "I snore a lot, and I'm tired all day." And if you just mention the words "sleep apnoea" it may trigger a light bulb. Doctors know about it, but, as I say, it's not always on their radar.'

If your doctor suspects you have sleep apnoea you'll probably be referred to a specialist, either at a public hospital, or at a private clinic. A bit like PSA tests for prostate cancer, we're stepping into a political arena here. Funding for public health dictates that unless you have very severe sleep apnoea you won't get free treatment. They're more lenient if you're a truck or train or bus driver, or a pilot, but if you don't drive or fly for a living, you may have to fund treatment yourself.

'So what you think,' says Alex Bartle, 'is, "Well the hospital is not going to treat me, so it's not an issue." But it is an issue, it's a huge issue. It sort of tells people that they're okay, when they're really not okay. It's just they haven't got the funding to treat all the sleep apnoea that actually exists out there.'

What's likely to happen if you go to a sleep specialist? There will almost certainly be a sleep test. They used to involve being wired up in much the way you are for heart monitoring, but now it may be no more complex than putting on a wrist band, and attaching a clip to a finger, then having your sleep patterns fed into a monitor beside the bed.

Clinics around the country vary, as do the costs, so it'll be worthwhile checking costs in your area. A consultation and the test could cost around $500.

How you'll be treated depends on how serious your problem is. For mild sleep apnoea you may be given a device to put in your mouth called a mandibular advancement splint. If you're a former contact sport player, it will remind you of a double mouthguard, covering your top and bottom teeth. The aim of the splint is to bring your lower jaw forward which, in turn, should bring your tongue forward, keeping it

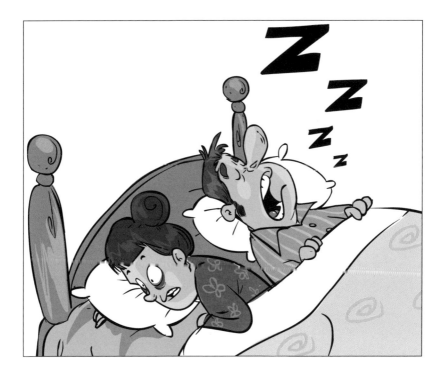

from falling back, blocking your throat and stopping you breathing.

'They're unobtrusive and quite small to carry around,' says Alex Bartle. 'But they're quite difficult to use. One of the downsides is that it can upset your jaw joint. That's what is called a temporomandibular joint, and it just stretches that because you're sleeping for eight hours or more with your jaw jutting forward.'

The gold standard for sleep apnoea treatment is a CPAP machine. CPAP stands for continuous positive airway pressure. It's a machine with a nose mask that you wear at night. While you sleep it feeds low-pressure air into your airways to keep them open.

Not everyone finds them easy to work at first, but, having used one for several years when I was very overweight, my experience was so good and dramatic it was a little like being touched by an angel. Not only did it stop the sleep apnoea I'd been diagnosed with, but it also stopped me snoring altogether. I'd tried the splint, which didn't have much effect at all. I'd even tried ridiculous little tapes on my nose that for a while were being used by rugby players because they were supposed to open your nostrils to help you breathe easier. For a while they were touted as helping sleep apnoea, but, as your nose plays no part in the problem, I might as well have gone to bed clutching a crystal.

The CPAP machine, which starts at around $1300 to buy, depending on the machine that's right for you, has a few downsides, but none of them are to do with the health benefits to you. The machine itself sits beside the bed, with tubes running to the nose mask. Your partner may take a while to adjust to the low hum it makes. You also, to be brutally honest, look a little like Hannibal Lecter when the mask's on.

But Alex Bartle makes an excellent point about the device. 'There's no question it looks odd. But nobody really sees it, because you only put it on when you turn out the light and say your goodnight. Then you're quiet, and that's what your partner wants; your partner doesn't care what you look like, just as long as in the dark you're quiet.'

I was one of about half the people who use a CPAP machine who found it easy to adjust to. Don't be spooked if it takes you a few weeks to get used to sleeping with one. It's enormously worthwhile to check that you have a therapist you can contact if you're having any difficulties using the machine. Once it's working you'll probably never stop. A survey by one private sleep clinic found that after a year more than 90% of people who had bought a machine were still using it every night.

Keep in mind that a CPAP machine doesn't cure sleep apnoea, but it will usually keep it under complete control. The benefits are many. For a start, you lose the symptoms (snoring, constantly feeling tired) and it reduces your risk of getting, or aggravating, high blood pressure, liver problems, and losing testosterone.

Another plus is that you'll probably find it easier to lose weight. Disturbed sleep changes your metabolism and makes you likely to eat more. Then added weight, combined with feeling tired, makes exercising much harder. For some people, removing the tiredness and the hunger may even see weight loss that leads to stopping snoring. If that doesn't happen the worst-case scenario is that you'll feel better, your partner will lead a happier, more restful life, and you'll have lowered the risk of other health problems.

There's a local website, <u>sleepapnoeanz.org.nz</u>, run by a voluntary organisation, and the Ministry of Health also recommends the site, <u>healthnavigator.org.nz/health-a-z/o/obstructive-sleep-apnoea</u>, which gives clear, helpful insights into the problem.

Sexual Health
Staying Well

When blues legend Robert Johnson sang about 'stones in my passway' in the 1930s it was a very subtle reference to gonorrhoea. By the time the 1970s rolled around and Dr Hook recorded a song called 'Penicillin Penny' there was very little confusion over what the lyrics meant.

What hasn't changed from the day in Dallas in 1937 when Johnson recorded his song is that the gold standard for preventing sexual diseases of all kinds is the condom. If you grew up in the 1960s condoms were a mysterious sexual aid, hidden under the counter at the chemist's, or surreptitiously dispensed by a barber after he dabbed talcum powder on your neck when he'd finished your short back and sides.

Shy Kiwi guys in past generations, too embarrassed to ask a young woman behind the counter at a chemist shop, would find themselves stockpiling toothpaste and Throaties cough lozenges because they couldn't bring themselves to say the word 'Durex' out loud. Today, of course, embarrassment about condoms is a thing of the past, as it should be. Condoms are on sale at every supermarket. At some high schools they're distributed free of charge.

So far, so sensible. The downside is when you only think of a condom as preventing pregnancy. And while it's true that unprotected sex with a woman in her mid-50s is unlikely to produce a baby, sexual diseases don't disappear with age. For a man having sex with a woman, or a man, a whole range of sexual infections are still out there.

An old joke once asked, 'Why are herpes and love different?'

The answer, 'Herpes is forever', is as true today as when herpes was a front-page topic for *Time* magazine in 1982. Drug companies have spent several fortunes looking for a cure, but so far without any luck, although it is now easily treated.

Gonorrhoea? Syphilis? Chlamydia? All still out there, at any age. HIV? Rates are actually increasing, especially in some groups.

Wait, wait, don't run away. If you're married, or in a long-term stable relationship, and only have one partner, your risk of sexual disease is negligible to zero says a sexually transmitted disease specialist, Rick Franklin. And there are now treatments that will cure, or, in the case of viral infections such as HIV, keep the infection at bay.

If you're a younger man, maybe under 30, there's a very good chance you'll have had sex education that includes making sure you use a condom, especially for new partners, or if you have more than one partner.

So how effective is a condom when it comes to sexual diseases?

'Like everything there is a degree of relativity going on here,' says Rick. 'So the condom will protect you way over 90% for penile vaginal sex. It is not often used, if ever, for things like oral sex which may also transmit infection. But in general, it is damn good protection. The condom is protective for both insertive forms of sex, be it anal or vaginal. You would want to use one for either of those activities.'

What about oral sex?

'The risks are lower. For heterosexual men and women having oral sex with each other, traditionally it has been pretty low risk. You can transmit infections by oral sex; gonorrhoea, for example, is often transmitted by oral sex. Chlamydia, not so much, but it can be. It's also very unlikely you'll catch HIV through oral sex. 'Genital herpes is classically transmitted by oral sex. Then again, once you get into an older grouping of men and women they have usually been exposed to those kinds of infections before. Not always, but usually.

'Oral sex contains a degree of risk. But for men it is lower than unprotected, penetrative sex.'

There's a slightly weird blip in condom use in recent years, and it can occur amongst older, heterosexual men, who have recently separated, or divorced, and are in new relationships.

'I think they struggle,' says Rick Franklin, 'because they weren't educated about sexual safety to the same level that the younger men are now. I think that men over 50 didn't use condoms when they were out doing whatever they were doing before they got married, or got into a regular relationship. Where, of course, now that would be a pretty sensible requirement if they were having sex with other partners, but they may not think of it.

'For example, I can think of 55-year-old guys who have been married for 20 years, and split up in the last 18 months or so. Somebody has pointed out to them that there's a social media app which allows them to find new partners astonishingly easily. Whereas in the past, it was never astonishingly easy for most men. There are a whole lot of so-called dating apps, but a lot of them are not dating apps at all, they are basically sex apps or hook-up apps. So when they get into that context, it is a bit like a kid in a candy shop, and they haven't had the social education around condom use. But condom use is what is required, because these are not partners who know each other's sexual history.'

If you're reading this and are worried about your sexual health, the tests are simple.

'The standard check-up at your GP would be a urine test, which tests for chlamydia and gonorrhoea, and a blood test, which would generally be looked at for syphilis and HIV, and perhaps hepatitis.'

Herpes? 'Unfortunately there is no simple screening test for herpes. But if there was something that is happening, like a sore or a blister on your penis, then go and get it checked. Go and get it checked!'

As with other forms of disease, early discovery is a huge help with the treatment of sexual infections, and they can all be treated, cured, or contained.

'If you're in the post-40, male heterosexual group, having partner change, and have had unprotected sex with new partners, then having regular check-ups and tests is a really good idea,' says Rick. 'It may save a whole lot of difficult and expensive problems.'

What is the current situation for gay men?

'We have been through this whole gambit of HIV,' says Rick, 'and I'm old enough, unfortunately, to have lived through the lot. AIDS came along [in the 1980s] and most patients who had HIV would die. There was very little you could do to save them. Then, slowly, pharmaceutical companies started producing drugs that helped, social awareness came along, and gay men banded together and started trying to figure out what the hell was going on, and why all their friends were dying. All these things were happening at the same time.

'Condom use became quite the norm and slowly drugs got better and better, and all those things combined led to a decrease in new infections. Then there was a kind of era when the drugs were good, treatments were much better, and men weren't dying of AIDS. But HIV infection rates have climbed steadily around the world from about the early or mid-2000s until now.

'Then along comes another change, and this new change is called PrEP. It stands for pre-exposure prophylaxis and treatment. The men who use this medication are not infected with HIV. They take the pills on a regular basis, usually five days out of seven. If they do that, they don't get infected, even if they have sex with a person who is HIV positive and not on treatment.

'So pre-exposure prophylaxis and treatment as prevention, where they have been introduced widely and with great support from the community and the government, can reduce new HIV infection rates. For example, in San Francisco for the last two years in a row the new HIV infection rates have decreased from the year before. Unheard of! If you told me that 10 years ago I would have laughed at you.'

As with many medical treatments in New Zealand, there's a political element at play here with PrEP. Ask Rick Franklin about PrEP, and he chooses his words carefully. Drug funding in this country is in the hands of a government-appointed body called Pharmac.

'This is not an anti-Pharmac rant,' says Rick, 'but for various reasons Pharmac is not a very liberal drug-funding organisation. New Zealand is a small country and drugs are very expensive. There is probably never going to be enough money in the public purse to do everything we wish to do. We still have limits on how soon we can start treatment for HIV, which is actually counterproductive. And we don't yet have funded pre-exposure prophylaxis.'

But Rick Franklin and his colleagues are involved in a small trial of pre-exposure prophylaxis with a grant from a drug company called Gilead who are providing the drug, called Truvada, free of charge.

'As with heterosexual men,' he says, 'condoms are still the social preventative gold standard, but unfortunately relying on their use alone has failed. If condoms alone were going to deliver us good results we wouldn't see a year on year increase in the rate of new HIV infection. And that is what we've seen around the world.

'Medical prevention, trying to find every person who is at risk of HIV, and testing them for HIV, and if they are positive, putting them immediately on treatment, plus pre-exposure prophylaxis, for those still negative, but at risk, combined with condoms, is the only thing that has led to a decrease in new infection.'

What's out there and how to deal with it

CHLAMYDIA *is a bacterial infection, the most common sexually trans-mitted infection in New Zealand, and in most countries around the world.*

The Cause: Having unprotected vaginal, anal or oral sex.
The Symptoms: In men there are either no symptoms, which is most likely, or it causes similar symptoms to gonorrhoea: a penal discharge and pain peeing. 'The majority don't have any symptoms at all,' says Rick. 'But in men it can be related to some deleterious long-term health effects, possibly infertility. It is certainly related to infertility in women, which is why it is such an important infection, which should be treated.'

How to Detect It: If you have had unprotected sex, a simple urine test will show whether you have chlamydia or not.

How to Fix It: A short course of antibiotics will usually completely cure chlamydia.

GONORRHOEA *is another bacterial infection.*

The Cause: It too can be caught from unprotected vaginal, anal or oral sex.

The Symptoms: There can be a white, green, or yellow discharge from the end of the penis, pain when peeing, sore testicles, irritation inside the penis, and discharge or bleeding from the anus.

How to Detect It: A urine test will confirm if you have it. Untreated it can lead to sterility.

How to Fix It: Gonorrhoea can be cured with antibiotics.

GENITAL HERPES *is caused by a virus called herpes simplex (HSV). There are two types, HSV-1, which causes cold sores around the mouth and genital and anal regions, and HSV-2 which causes infections in the genital and anal areas.*

The Cause: Oral sex and penetrative sex.

The Symptoms: If you contract genital herpes, you may not experience any symptoms for months, years, or possibly not for the rest of your life. On the other hand, you may have symptoms as soon as two days after contracting the disease. Those may include itching, tingling, burning or pain in the genital area, painful spots or sores that become fluid-filled blisters, a redness or a rash around the genital area, swelling, pain when peeing, and flu-like symptoms.

How to Detect It: A test from a suspicious lesion will usually detect genital herpes. Blood tests are generally not helpful.

How to Fix It: There is no cure. The main treatment is usually an anti-viral drug that will usually help speed up recovery from an outbreak, and reduce the number of times outbreaks occur.

SYPHILIS *is a bacterial disease.*

The Cause: Unprotected vaginal, anal or oral sex.

The Symptoms: It usually first appears as a small, painless sore. It may be on the penis, or hidden in your anus or mouth. Untreated the sore, called a chancre, will heal, but the syphilis has not been cured. A rash, usually non-itchy, may start on your torso, and might eventually cover most of your body. Untreated syphilis can go to a latent, or hidden, stage, until, in about 15 to 30% of cases, it reappears some years later, causing damage to the brain, nerves, eyes, heart, blood vessels, liver, bones, and joints. In New Zealand, says Rick Franklin, there has been a resurgence in syphilis, with cases increasing by more than 200% in the last five years. 'That has been driven by men having sex with men, but if you have a lot of syphilis amongst men having sex with men, there will be some of those men who are bisexual, and they will have sex with women as well.' Some of those women will catch syphilis, and then there's a danger, if they have a baby, of congenital syphilis, which can lead to many serious complications for the baby, including deafness. In both men and women untreated syphilis can damage internal organs so badly it can eventually result in death.

How to Detect It: A blood test.

How to Fix It: In the early stages it can be easily treated, usually with penicillin, which kills the organism that causes syphilis. If found at a later stage, treatment with penicillin may take longer.

HIV (Human Immunodeficiency Virus) *is, as the full name sug-gests, a virus.*

The Cause: HIV can only be caught through the bloodstream; that is, via infectious fluids entering your bloodstream. Many more gay men than heterosexual men in New Zealand have HIV. In 2015 there were 153 men diagnosed with HIV who had sex with other men, while 24 men were diagnosed with HIV after sex with women. Gay men are more susceptible because if you have anal intercourse you are 18 times more likely to contract HIV than from vaginal intercourse. The Aids Foundation of New Zealand urges men who have anal intercourse to wear a condom and use a lube, which will dramatically reduce risk.

The Symptoms: They can include fatigue, weight loss, and flu-like symptoms. But often HIV will have no symptoms for months, or as long as 10 years. If HIV is untreated the final stage is AIDS (Acquired Immunodeficiency Syndrome). AIDS is the last stage of HIV, reducing the body's immune system's ability to fight off infection and disease.

How to Detect It: A blood test, which may literally be lifesaving.

How to Fix It: Drug treatment for HIV has improved so much since the early 1990s that Rick Franklin says, 'If a man came to see me and we sat down and we had a conversation about the fact that he had recently been diagnosed with HIV, then I tell him that in most cases, if he takes his medications regularly, and gets appropriate medical care, his life expectancy should be close to normal for his age. So that is way different from what we were talking about when HIV and Aids first appeared.'

A good first stop online is again health.govt.nz, the Ministry of Health website. Click on 'Your Health' on the home page, and individual sexual diseases will appear on a list of general diseases. For more specific, highly practical, advice about HIV and Aids, the Aids Foundation website, at nzaf.org.nz, is a great resource.

How to Be a Mate
& Other Hints For Life

As a 16-year-old starting an apprenticeship as a butcher Peter Leitch could never have dreamed the day would come when he'd be a knighted national icon. He built the Mad Butcher chain to 16 stores before selling the company in 2007. He's always been involved in charity work, organising luncheons that raised as much as $145,000 a time. He's now the Patron and Honorary Ambassador of New Zealand Rugby League, Auckland Rugby League, the Vodafone Warriors, Allergy NZ, Diabetes Auckland, The Prostate Cancer Foundation of NZ, and Macular Degeneration NZ. And he's the 19th Vodafone Warrior. Most importantly, from the time when he was a young, struggling butcher and gave his local Mangere East league club meat packs to raffle, he's always been a kind, generous man. He shares his thoughts on friendship, business, ethics and sport.

On being a mate

I have a saying that is really simple: The greatest gift you can give anyone is your time. People take time for granted. A lot of people say that I'm a very generous man, but that's bullshit. I am not a billionaire so I can't give money away like water.

I have done what I can, but the one thing that I am proud of is I have given a lot of time to people. For example, I have a friend in hospital, Rodney Green. I go in there every day to see him. Every day. No matter how much pressure I was under, I still went in to see him. And that is the greatest gift you can give anyone.

The pleasure of giving

I genuinely like making people happy. There are two things about that: A) I love people, and B) I like making them happy. I get great enjoyment from it.

I give my card out many times. Let's say I meet a kid in Warrior gear, I'll say, 'You email me and I'll send you something.' It may only be a book or posters or something. They get a buzz out of it.

In Queenstown there was a kid with a Warriors jersey and he came from Western Australia. They were his favourite team, so I sent him a poster. I got an email the other day from his father thanking me; he just couldn't believe it.

Does it do your own soul good? I'm not sure about that, but it's a great moment when someone feels happy. I did something for Diabetes New Zealand the other day with Monty Betham, and they drove me there and back. As we drove along the road there was a Maori guy in a wheelchair on the side of the road, and I sung out, 'Gidday bro, how you going mate?' And his eyes lit up, 'Oh, the Mad Butcher!' I get a real thrill out of that.

Saying thanks

I think a simple thank you is very important. Being polite is always a good idea. For example, sometimes people email me, or get in touch through Facebook, asking for a donation, and they just send a standard letter. They don't go the extra mile and make it personal.

Last week I rang a lady from Dunedin whose young boy has got cancer, and they were looking for some prizes to fundraise. She'd sent me a letter. It had no 'How are you, Mr Leitch?' No nothing. I rang her and I said, 'Please don't take this the wrong way, I'm trying to teach you something.' I said, 'It would have been nice if you had addressed the letter to me, "Dear Sir Peter" or "Dear Butch". Firstly, "How are you? I hope you are well. We are having a fundraiser, can you help us?"'

She took it on board. She sent me an email back, and said thanks for the advice, it's good.

Always reply

This is strange, sometimes I have to ring people and turn them down, and they thank me because I've got back to them. A lot of people don't get back to them, you see. I make a point of trying to get back to everyone. Being polite again.

Get the money

If you're putting on a function as a charity fundraiser, make sure you actually sell the tickets before the fundraiser. Don't rely on people paying at the door.

It's very important, because talk is cheap. Action is what's required. Until you've got the money in the bank, the tickets aren't sold.

When you have a function you have to pay for the catering. Say you are going to have a luncheon for 200 people, you have got to pay for 200 people. If only 100 turn up, half of the money you are raising has gone already, because you still have to pay the caterers.

Trust in business

Trust means a lot in business and I got some good deals, very good deals, because people knew I would pay the bill. In business it is okay for Phil Gifford to say he'll give you more for the product than Peter Leitch would, but if Phil Gifford is not going to pay the bill you are getting nothing. You can't buy honesty. You can't buy integrity.

A butcher before a businessman

My claim to fame in business is that I started a chain that has had 35 or so shops. Compared to someone like Michael Hill I wasn't a great businessman, but I do believe I was a good butcher who knew what people wanted, good meat at reasonable prices, and I gave them that.

I got on because I wheeled and dealed. I didn't have a big bank balance, I didn't have rich parents. So I had to use my skills as a trader. You do me a favour, I'll do you a favour.

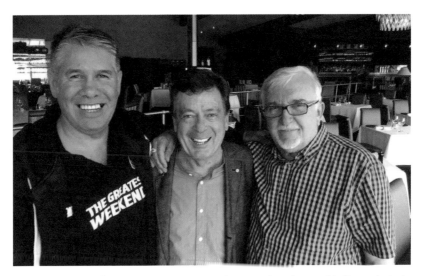

'The greatest gift you can give anyone is your time,' says Sir Peter Leitch.
Two men who return the favour are, on left, policeman and closest mate,
Dexter Traill, and, centre, award-winning radio host Leighton Smith.

Being loyal

It would be fair to say I always try to reward loyalty with loyalty. I never forget if someone's been fair and decent to me.

Working hard

That's one thing I wasn't scared of: hard work. I had three jobs when I opened my first shop. I was working from daylight to dusk. I've got to be honest, there were times when I thought, 'Shit, is this worth it?' But in retirement it is certainly worth it. I don't have to worry. We're not billionaires, but we are in a very safe financial space.

On losing in sport

Sometimes if the Warriors or the Kiwis lose I have people say to me, 'What a tragedy, you must be really upset.' I always reply, 'Did anyone die? Was a child hurt?' Because if that didn't happen it's not a tragedy, it's a football game we lost.

Aging
Forever Young

The golden years. In this country at 65 you even get a gold card so you know exactly when they start. There can be a lot more to them than travelling free on buses. It just takes a bit of planning.

Many of us plan financially. Sometimes for decades and decades ahead, sometimes without even doing much ourselves. Look at KiwiSaver, which is specifically aimed at making life more comfortable for someone who'll retire in 30 or 40 years. There's a good government website for financial planning for later in life called sorted.org.nz.

But there's more to retirement than balancing your books, as important as that may be. Your bank account can't talk with you, go out for a meal with you, or watch the footy and cheer or groan about it. By sheer good luck, and how smart women are about their health, just because you're a man, when you hit 75, there's about a 75% chance you won't be living alone. Your wife or partner will still be alive. On the other hand, nearly half of 75-year-old women will be on their own.

And better still, if you've worked out ways to stay socially connected, you'll not only be healthier, but you'll also live longer. That's not just word-of-mouth folk wisdom. Researchers at the University of California, San Francisco, recently kept tabs for six years on 1600 people, whose average age was 71 when the study started. Participants who said they weren't lonely were less likely to develop difficulties coping with daily living. And there was a huge difference in mortality rates. Of those who said they didn't feel lonely, just 14% had passed away within six years, compared to 23% who reported being lonely.

So how do you go about making your life happier, longer and more satisfying? Having a plan to keep active and healthy will be worth every minute spent. Joe Singh, a geriatrician on Auckland's North Shore, who has worked with elderly people since 1987, says there are basic but important areas to consider. Loneliness, he says, 'can be a bugger when you're old'.

One area to look at is keeping reasonably physically fit. And an important side effect of staying active can be that it helps you make sure you don't become socially isolated. Joe himself plays tennis and squash on a regular basis. 'It allows you to meet different people and grow old with them. There are people of various ages who play with us, some up to 80 years old, but they like it, and come along two to three times a week because it not only has physical advantages but it's a social outing too.'

Keeping social contacts up, he believes, keeps people healthier. 'There's certainly less depression.'

If you're still working, and look in the mirror and start to see grey winning the battle of the hair colour, for God's sake don't just reach for the dye bottle. Ask any woman to answer honestly and she'll tell you a 70-year-old with jet-black hair looks even more like a 70-year-old! Instead, give yourself the gift of a quiet time to figure out just what you want to do when you're not heading for work after breakfast.

One good idea might be to ask mates who have retired what they did, what they enjoyed, and what they wouldn't have done if they'd known better. Start thinking hard about what you like, and what you might enjoy sharing with other people. It will take a bit of work. But the effort will be worth it.

It's startling how many organisations there are out there to help you connect with others. If you log into a site called meetup.com you'll find that in Auckland, for example, there are groups, not age specific, looking for people to do everything from watching sports events together, to playing social table tennis, to doing nude yoga (by the way, it is legit, and they sternly warn they're tough on 'inappropriate behaviour').

The important thing is to do what makes you happy. Staying in touch with what's happening in the world is good for you too, says Joe Singh. Talking with your partner or friends about what you read in the paper, or what you saw on the news, is valuable. Technically, it's called 'reality orientation', which is basically being up to speed with what's happening in the world.

Part of that world now is the net, which Joe feels offers older people a great means of not only keeping up to date with news and society, but is also a way to communicate with family and friends, as we become a more mobile society, with kids and grandkids often living in different cities or towns or overseas.

You'll also often find, says Joe, that your doctor may suggest sites to visit online that can give more details of something you're being treated for. 'I'm talking about the British Medical Association site, or the New Zealand Diabetes Foundation, not a chat site that says "stop all medicines today". That's your choice, but it's probably not helpful.'

So it becomes important, if you're considering moving into a retirement village or home, to make sure one item on the checklist is whether WiFi is available.

'For a lot of guys, I'd also be looking to see if they have Sky, so you can watch sport on TV.'

Old-school ways can keep your brain active too.

'It might be Sudoku, or crosswords, or jigsaw puzzles, but I think that kind of mental stimulation is important, and it's good to engage in on a daily basis, which will keep your brain going.'

Then there's keeping an eye on your general health.

'Men traditionally are not very good at getting regular health checks. There's a bit of a "she'll be right" attitude, and men often wait until a problem has really manifested before they see a doctor. Visit your doctor once a year. After 65, I don't think that's overdoing it at all. It really should be the minimum.

'It's a funny thing, but when you actually get to your doctor's appointment, you sometimes start talking about things that you hadn't thought were important, like having a little shortness of breath when you go up the stairs.

'A problem with men, a lot more than with women, can be that they put a lot of things down to, "Oh, I'm just getting old." For example, with Parkinson's disease we can see diagnosis delayed, because it comes on gradually, and people start to walk slowly, generally do things more slowly. And they say, "Well, that's part of aging," until they walk in here and it's obvious they have Parkinson's. And that's manageable but, like almost all things, the sooner it's treated the better.

'There's a problem called polymyalgia, which is basically aches and pains in the muscles that come on. It's a very treatable condition, that absolutely gets back to normal if you pick it up early, but people can go two or three months thinking that they've just got aches and pains from excessive gardening, or making some excuse of getting older, when really they're harbouring something that's quite treatable.

'With some things, you can look fine, but with blood pressure and blood tests, early markers can be found, and conditions treated.'

The net as a friend

The net — or, as an old mate in radio used to call it, 'this interweb thing' — is a great eye on the world. You can read newspapers and magazines online, keep in touch with family and friends, find phone numbers, and even track down a song you haven't heard for 50 years, and listen to it for free. But if you didn't grow up with the net, here are a few tips that'll make sure it doesn't sting you:

If a Nigerian princess sends an email wanting help, and offers to pay you millions of dollars if you'll just send a trifling few thousand to her bank account to cover bank fees, it's a lie. Ignore it.

If a lawyer you've never heard of sends you an email saying you've inherited a large sum from a relative you've never heard of, and just wants your bank account details to transfer the money to, it's a lie. Ignore it.

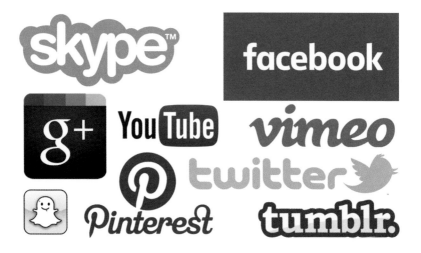

If a nice man or woman rings you and says they're from Microsoft, and have detected a problem with your computer, and needs your passwords to fix it, then it's a lie. Hang up.

If Kitty from Hong Kong sends an email saying she's seen you online, and has fallen in love with you, it's a lie. Ignore it.

In fact, if anyone you don't know offers you money or love, or both, in return for money and/or personal details, I'm sorry, but it's a lie.

On the other hand, here are sites that are genuine, and offer good ideas:

Sorted.org.nz is a government site that offers financial advice. It's not designed to get you to put savings with a specific organisation, so you can trust what you read.

Meetup.com sounds like a dating site, but it's not. It feeds instead into numerous groups in your area that are open to new members.

Ageconcern.org.nz has been around since 1948 (when it began in Dunedin as the Otago Old People's Welfare Council, the name changing in 1991), and the site offers advice on everything from housing and nutrition, to explaining how to access a visiting service to ease social isolation.

AN OLD GUY'S JOKE

Two mates, John and Gary, both in their late 70s, haven't caught up for several months, when they bump into each other at the dairy.

Gary says, 'What's new in your life?'

'I got married three months ago,' says John.

'Nice woman?'

'No, not really. Pretty grumpy actually.'

'Oh. I suppose she must have the looks to make up for it.'

'No, I wouldn't say she's pretty.'

There's a pause. 'Is she wealthy then?'

'No. Her last husband died without leaving her a cent.'

'Okay. Look, I don't want to be crude, but is she good in bed?'

John laughs. 'Mate, we've got separate bedrooms. There's no sex involved.'

Gary's now really bemused. 'So she's grumpy, unattractive, poor and there's no romance. Why the hell did you marry her?'

'She can still drive at night.'

Picking Your Coach

Think of a visit to your doctor (your general practitioner or GP) as being similar to the mentoring role Wayne Smith was asked to take on a few years ago with Beauden Barrett.

Barrett was starting to find himself caught too often when he went to run with the ball. Smith spotted small telltale signs Barrett was making, some always before he attacked, some always before he kicked. They'd been picked up by video analysts in Super rugby. Defenders would then be one tiny, but vital, step ahead of Barrett when he had the ball. Barrett made slight changes suggested by Smith and, as so many floundering international defenders will now tell you, has never looked back.

Going to the doctor isn't the adult version of being called to the headmaster's office. You're not on trial. It's not a test that if you fail will lead to punishment. If seeing your doctor feels like a test, or a trial to you, find a new doctor.

If you don't have a doctor, ask a friend, or a family member, or a workmate, what their doctor's like. Ring the surgery of whoever gets the thumbs up.

Because even if you've been healthy enough to get through life without ever having a GP, there are huge benefits for you in having one. Why is that? Having a doctor who knows you means you've got the equivalent of the coach who has a baseline to work from, and will notice changes. Because he or she knows what's needed for you to stay well, and will let you know just how to do that. A doctor who sees you regularly will make a range of tests, keep the results, and instantly spot any early-warning signs if something changes.

Not only will your doctor help you stay fitter, and enjoy everything you do a bit more, he or she might actually save your life, because the best specialists in the world are no use if you never get to see them.

So if you take only one piece of advice from this book, please, PLEASE make it this:

SIGN UP WITH A DOCTOR. NOW!

About the Author

PHIL GIFFORD has won nine New Zealand and two Australasian radio awards, has twice been judged New Zealand sportswriter of the year, and three times New Zealand sports columnist of the year. He has won two Dulux national print awards for news reporting, in 1976 (on the *Capitaine Bougainville* shipwreck) and 1981 (on the Springbok tour). He writes a column in the *Sunday Star-Times,* and a music column in *North & South* magazine. He is a weekly member of 'The Panel' on 'Veitch On Sport', and 'The Sports Huddle' on the Larry Williams show on NewstalkZB. Phil has worked at every World Cup since 1987. He has been a Television ONE sports newsreader, fronted the shows *That's Fairly Interesting* and *Don't Tell Me,* and was an original panel member on *Game of Two Halves.* He was a scriptwriter for Billy T James' television shows, and co-wrote the script for the 2011 feature film on James' life, *Te Movie.* He invented the satirical rugby character Loosehead Len in 1973, and wrote the columns for 32 years. In 2010 he was honoured with the SPARC lifetime achievement award for services to sports journalism. He has written 25 books. His memoir *Loose Amongst the Legends* was named as one of the biographies of the year in the *Listener* magazine's 100 best books of 2014. He lives in Auckland with his wife Jan.